C000151061

Risk factors for amputation in patient

Nikhil Nanjappa
Tirou Aroul
Robinson Smile

Risk factors for amputation in patients with diabetic foot ulcers

Based on a perspective study of 120 patients at a tertiary care hospital in India for over 20 years

LAP LAMBERT Academic Publishing

Impressum/Imprint (nur für Deutschland/only for Germany)
Bibliografische Information der Deutschen Nationalbibliothek: Die Deutsche Nationalbibliothek verzeichnet diese Publikation in der Deutschen Nationalbibliografie; detaillierte bibliografische Daten sind im Internet über http://dnb.d-nb.de abrufbar.
Alle in diesem Buch genannten Marken und Produktnamen unterliegen warenzeichen-, marken- oder patentrechtlichem Schutz bzw. sind Warenzeichen oder eingetragene Warenzeichen der jeweiligen Inhaber. Die Wiedergabe von Marken, Produktnamen, Gebrauchsnamen, Handelsnamen, Warenbezeichnungen u.s.w. in diesem Werk berechtigt auch ohne besondere Kennzeichnung nicht zu der Annahme, dass solche Namen im Sinne der Warenzeichen- und Markenschutzgesetzgebung als frei zu betrachten wären und daher von jedermann benutzt werden dürften.

Coverbild: www.ingimage.com

Verlag: LAP LAMBERT Academic Publishing GmbH & Co. KG
Heinrich-Böcking-Str. 6-8, 66121 Saarbrücken, Deutschland
Telefon +49 681 3720-310, Telefax +49 681 3720-3109
Email: info@lap-publishing.com

Approved by: SRI BALAJI VIDYAPEETH UNIVERSITY, Diss, 2009

Herstellung in Deutschland (siehe letzte Seite)
ISBN: 978-3-659-15264-1

Imprint (only for USA, GB)
Bibliographic information published by the Deutsche Nationalbibliothek: The Deutsche Nationalbibliothek lists this publication in the Deutsche Nationalbibliografie; detailed bibliographic data are available in the Internet at http://dnb.d-nb.de.
Any brand names and product names mentioned in this book are subject to trademark, brand or patent protection and are trademarks or registered trademarks of their respective holders. The use of brand names, product names, common names, trade names, product descriptions etc. even without a particular marking in this works is in no way to be construed to mean that such names may be regarded as unrestricted in respect of trademark and brand protection legislation and could thus be used by anyone.

Cover image: www.ingimage.com

Publisher: LAP LAMBERT Academic Publishing GmbH & Co. KG
Heinrich-Böcking-Str. 6-8, 66121 Saarbrücken, Germany
Phone +49 681 3720-310, Fax +49 681 3720-3109
Email: info@lap-publishing.com

Printed in the U.S.A.
Printed in the U.K. by (see last page)
ISBN: 978-3-659-15264-1

Copyright © 2012 by the author and LAP LAMBERT Academic Publishing GmbH & Co. KG and licensors
All rights reserved. Saarbrücken 2012

CONTENTS

<u>ACKNOWLEDGEMENT</u>

The authors would like to take this opportunity to thank *Prof. D R GUNASEKARAN*, **Vice-Chancellor, Shri Balaji Vidyapeeth University**, for his unparalleled guidance, unwavering support, and constant inspiration towards the completion of this dissertation.

We would like to thank the Dean of **Mahatma Gandhi Medical College & Research Institute,** *Prof. G. MUTHURANGAN* and the management team of Sri Balaji Vidyapeeth University for their constant support and encouragement.

We would like to thank, *Prof. N ANANTHAKRISHNAN*, Coordinator of post graduate studies, for lending his expertise towards writing of this dissertation.

The authors would like to thank all the faculty of department of surgery for their guidance and support all along.

We want to thank *MR. LOKESHMARAN* for lending his expertize for the statistical analysis.

The authors would like to thank their families for their love and support.

I would like to express my gratitude to all the *nursing and the housekeeping* staff of MGMCRI for their help in patient care.

The authors would like to thank all the patients, who volunteered to be a part of this study.

INTRODUCTION

Diabetic foot ulcer is a rising health problem with rising prevalence of diabetes. It is the most important cause of non-traumatic foot amputations. Diabetic foot ulcers are primarily due to neuropathy and / or ischemia, which are frequently complicated by infection. Throughout the world, foot lesions and foot infections are the leading causes of hospitalization and prolonged hospital stays in diabetic patients.

Up to 85% of all diabetic foot related problems are preventable through a combination of good foot care and appropriate education for patients and health care providers. The holistic care of a diabetic foot ulcer needs a multidisciplinary approach. Apart from blood sugar control, treatment of ulcer involves debridement, offloading, appropriate dressings, vascular maintenances and infection control. Use of adjunctive treatments such as various growth factors, skin replacement dressings and vacuum assisted closure will accelerate healing in selected cases.

Lower extremity amputation is one of the most feared complications of diabetes. There are multiple risk factors which if co-exist in a patient delays the healing of the foot ulcer and in most patients leads to limb threatening and life threatening conditions which invariably progress to amputation of the lower extremity. The single most important factor in preventing amputation is detailed and repeated education of the patient in foot care. In our study we are evaluating the risk factors which lead to lower extremity amputation in diabetic foot.

REVIEW OF LITERATURE

Diabetes is one of the oldest diseases known to mankind. The Ebers Papyrus of 1500 B.C. mentions its symptoms and suggests treatment. However, the history of gangrene of the foot goes back to Biblical time, when, in Chronicles II, the first case of gangrene of the feet, perhaps due to diabetes, is described. The relationship between diabetic neuropathy, the insensitive foot, and foot ulceration was recognized by Pryce, a British surgeon, over a century ago. He stated that, "It was abundantly evident that the actual cause of the perforating ulcer was peripheral nerve degeneration and that diabetes itself played an active part in the causation of the perforating ulcer" [1]. Diabetic foot is especially vulnerable to amputation because of the frequent complications of peripheral neuropathy (PN), infection and peripheral arterial disease (PAD). A combination of this triad leads to the final cataclysmic events, gangrene and amputation. Fifty percent of all non-traumatic amputations are performed on the diabetics.

Fifteen percent of all diabetics will develop a foot ulcer during their lifetime [2]. Most of these are a result of peripheral neuropathy and the insensate foot which leads to painless trauma and ulceration. Diabetic foot problems are a major cause of hospitalization and prolonged hospital stays. Twenty percent of all diabetic persons who enter the hospital do so because of foot problems [3]. In the series of Smith et al, foot problems were responsible for 23% of the hospital days over a two-year period [4]. At the Indian Institute of Diabetes in Bombay, India, more than 10% of all admissions for diabetes are primarily for foot problems. More than 70% required surgical intervention and in more 40% of those interventions there was a toe or limb amputation [5]. In the U.K, more than 50% of bed occupancy of diabetics is due to foot problems [6]. It is obvious from these figures that throughout the world diabetic foot problems are a major cause of hospitalization, morbidity and mortality.

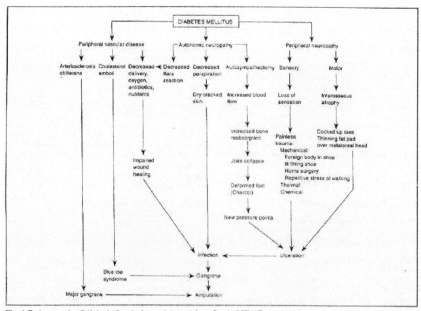

Fig. 1 Pathogenesis of diabetic foot lesions. Adapted from Levin ME. "Pathogenesis and management of diabetic foot lesions" In Levin ME, O'Neal LW, and Bowker JH, eds. The Diabetic Foot, 5th ed. St. Louis, Mosby Year-Book, 1993.

ETIOLOGY OF DIABETIC FOOT PROBLEMS

The main underlying risk factors for foot ulcers in diabetic patients are peripheral neuropathy and ischemia.

NEUROPATHY

Epidemiologic studies have found that the point prevalence of distal lower limb neuropathy ranges from 30% to 50% of the diabetic population studied [7, 8]. Both type 1 and type 2 diabetic patients are similarly affected. With such frequent occurrence of neuropathy, it is no surprise that more than 60% of diabetic patients' foot ulcers are primarily due to underlying neuropathy [9] . The distal neuropathy of diabetes affects all components of the nervous system: sensory, motor, and autonomic, each of which contributes to foot ulcer development. Loss of nerve function correlates with chronic hyperglycemia, as reflected in the mean level of glycosylated hemoglobin over time [10]. Ischemia of the endoneurial microvascular circulation induced by metabolic abnormalities, from hyperglycemia is believed to be the underlying mechanism for nerve degeneration[11, 12].

Motor nerve involvement & deformities

Loss of neural supply to the intrinsic muscles of the foot produces an imbalance of the long flexor and extensor tendons. Contraction of the more powerful flexors of the lower limb induces the classic high-arched foot and claw toe deformity seen in as many as 50% of patients with diabetes [13.] Hyperextension of the toes with resultant overriding of the metatarsal-phalangeal joints forces the metatarsal heads downward, thereby increasing their prominence. Hyperextension of the toes displaces the metatarsal fat pads distally, further reducing the natural cushioning of the metatarsal heads. These mechanical changes increase plantar pressures inducing callus formation and underlying skin breakdown. Splaying of the foot from loss of the intrinsic muscles, in combination with disruption of the normal bony relationship of the distal foot, culminates in the foot that is wider and thicker than normal. Shoes that once fit that patient therefore no longer fit. Ill-fitting shoes cause areas of local trauma.

Autonomic neuropathy & ulceration

Autonomic dysfunction of the foot from diabetic neuropathy results in loss of sweat and oil gland function. Anhidrosis leads to dry, fissured skin susceptible to bacterial invasion. Furthermore, loss of peripheral sympathetic vascular tone in the lower limb increases distal arterial flow and pressure, which, by damaging the capillary basement membrane, might contribute to peripheral edema. Edema increases the risk of foot ulceration by adding another element of minor trauma caused by wearing shoes that fit even more poorly as the edema increases.

Sensory neuropathy:

The motor and autonomic neural abnormalities would have far less effect were it not for the concurrent loss of protective sensation in the foot. Normally, if the foot developed a fissure of blister, or if bony structure changed, patients would feel the discomfort and take appropriate corrective measures. Unfortunately, with onset of the peripheral neuropathy of diabetes, this protective response diminishes and can eventually disappear with progressive reduction in nerve function. This sequence of events allows patients to walk with apparent comfort on ever-deepening ulcers. The lack of pain lulls patients, and often physicians, into a false sense of security, a misguided "but it doesn't hurt; therefore it cannot be a serious problem".

ISCHEMIA

The other major underlying cause of diabetic foot ulcers is peripheral vascular disease. Primarily ischemic ulcer without substantial accompanying neuropathy accounts for approximately 15% to 20% of foot ulcers, and another 15% to 20% have a mixed neuropathic-vascular etiology [9]. Overall, atherosclerosis of the lower limbs in people with diabetes occurs at least two or three times more often than in people without diabetes and has a predilection for affecting the tibial and peroneal arteries of the calf with relative sparing of the arteries of the foot [14,15]. This pattern differs from the general population, where more proximal atherosclerotic changes predominate. Involvement of the peripheral autonomic nervous system has been proposed to explain the more distal distribution of lower limb atherosclerosis among diabetic patients. Autonomic dysfunction reduces the normal vasoconstriction that occurs in the lower leg arteries with standing and results in the increase in the intra luminal flow and pressure that is aggravated by gravitational forces [16]. Reduced vasoconstrictive ability further reduces vessels' capacity to expand in response to systolic pressure. The combination of high flow and reduced wall motion encourages formation of plaque in calf arteries [17]. Interestingly, among diabetic patients, smoking does not seem to be associated with recurrent foot ulcers or risk of amputation from ischemia [18,19]. These data conflict with information about patients without diabetes, which clearly indicates that smoking is a risk factor for claudication and amputation [20]. Regardless of whether smoking affects lower limb complications, diabetic patients who smoke have all mortality twice that of non-smoking diabetic patients and should be strongly counseled to end cigarette smoking [21.]

SPECIAL DIABETIC FOOT PROBLEMS

The Heel

The heel of the diabetic patient is particularly vulnerable to trauma. When as diabetic patient is required to have bed rest for any length of time, such as when hospitalized, particular attention must be paid to the heel. Because of loss of sensation, the patient tends to keep the heels in the same position. This results in pressure necrosis causing the skin to break down. Infection and gangrene can follow. These patients should have their heels inspected at least once and preferably twice a day. If erythema is present, aggressive protective intervention must be instituted. Prevention is critical. This is best achieved by turning the patient, using heel protectors, and an air suspension mattress. The available heel protectors may not stay in place; therefore frequent checks are required.

Foot Deformities

Foot deformities frequently lead to ulceration. Diabetics are particularly prone to develop cocked up toes which can result in pressure at the top of the tip of the toes. This is referred as the "tip-top-toe syndrome" [22]. This deformity is frequently associated with a thinning or shifting of the fat pad under the first metatarsal head. These areas, the tops and tips of the toes, and the area under the first metatarsal head are therefore very vulnerable to ulceration and infection. The ideal treatment is prophylactic surgery to straighten these toes while the circulation is still good. When prophylactic surgery cannot be carried out, these patients should wear a shoe with a larger toe box or an in-depth shoe with a cushioned insole to protect the toes and metatarsal head area.

Bunions are common and frequently lead to ulceration and infection. Prophylactic surgery is the ideal treatment.

The Charcot foot is the classic diabetic foot deformity. The Charcot foot develops in four stages. In the first or acute stage the patient usually presents with a history of mild trauma and a hot, red, swollen foot with bounding pulses. This must be differentiated from cellulitis. Once infection has been ruled out and a diagnosis of Charcot foot has been established, the treatment is non-weight bearing. This is best accomplished with a contact cast. If the patient is allowed to ambulate, the second stage of the Charcot foot develops, with the beak down of the bones of the foot, resulting in fractures. The x-ray at the time of the patient's initial visit may be perfectly normal. Calcification of the interosseous arteries is rarely found. The second stage develops in a two to three week interval. Repeat x-ray may show fractures, usually at the tarso-metatarsal joint but not infrequently at the distal ends of the metatarsals. The third stage of the Charcot foot is characterized by foot deformity. The foot takes on a club foot appearance or a rocker bottom configuration. Treatment at this stage requires the use of special molded shoes. If the patient continues to walk on unprotected feet, the fourth stage ensues with development of a plantar ulceration in the area of the arch. The ulceration can become infected, leading to gangrene and amputation [23].

EXERCISE FOR DIABETICS WITH FOOT PROBLEMS

Exercise is an important modality in the management of diabetes. However, in-patients with PAD and PN, weight bearing exercises such as jogging, prolonged walking, treadmill, and step exercises may need to be curtailed or avoided. The presence of an active foot ulcer is an absolute contraindication for weight bearing exercise. Patients who have a healed ulcer must take special precautions when exercising. Scar tissue is not good tissue and is vulnerable to the sheer forcers of walking. Patients with PAD, PN and an insensate foot can do a variety of non-weight bearing exercises such as swimming, bicycling, rowing, chair and upper body exercises. Diabetic persons, particularly those with PAD, PN and previously healed ulcerations, should have specific and detailed instructions in foot care and techniques for decreasing foot pressure before undertaking an exercise program. Physical therapists and personnel in exercise centers should discuss with the referring physicians the type of exercise program suitable for the diabetic.

CLASSIFICATION OF FOOT ULCERS

Meggitt-Wagner Classification

*Grade 0: High risk foot ulcer

*Grade 1: Superficial ulcer, not clinically infected

*Grade 2: Deep ulcer, often with cellulites

*Grade 3: Deep ulcer with bony involvement or abscess formation

*Grade 4: Localized gangrene (toe, forefoot or heel)

*Grade 5: Gangrene of the whole foot.

University Of Texas Classification

Grade lesion on depth first:

*Grade 0: No open ulcer or deformity

*Grade 1: Superficial ulcer

*Grade 2: penetration to tendon or joint capsule

*Grade 3: Penetrates to bone or joint space

After grading, then stage:

*Stage A: No infection or ischemia

*Stage B: With infection

*Stage C: With ischemia

*Stage D: Ischemia and infection present

University Of Texas Classification is better than Wagner Classification [24].

Table 1
Management of diabetic foot ulcers

I.   A. Evaluation
     B. Depth of penetration
     C. X-ray
          1. Foreign body
          2. Osteomyelitis
          3. Subcutaneous gas
     D. Location
     E. Biopsy
     F. Blood supply (non-invasive vascular studies)
II. Debridement, radical
III. Bacterial cultures (aerobic and anaerobic)
IV. Metabolic control
V.   Antibiotics
     A. Oral
     B. Parenteral
VI. Do not soak feet
VII. Decrease oedema
VIII.No weight bearing
     A. Bed rest
     B. Crutches
     C. Wheelchair
     D. Contact casting
IX. Improve circulation (vascular surgery)

Adapted from Levin ME. "Pathogenesis and management of diabetic foot lesions" In Levin ME, O'Neal LW, and Bowker JH, eds. The Diabetic Foot, 5th ed., St. Louis, Mosby Year-Book, 1993.

Table 1: Lists the steps in the management of diabetic foot ulcer 25. X-rays are necessary to rule out osteomyelitis, gas formation, the presence of foreign objects and asymptomatic fractures. Ideally any foot with ulceration or infection should be x rayed.

Treatment of a foot ulcer requires establishment of depth and degree of ulceration. What appears to be a superficial ulceration may be only the tip of the iceberg. There may be penetration deep into tissues. Vigorous debridement of the ulcer must be done to establish the degree of penetration and to remove all necrotic tissue. Debridement should be carried out upto healthy tissue. The ulcer following debridement will, in all probability, be larger than it was at presentation. Eschars should be completely removed. Whirlpool is not the method of choice for debridement. When the foot is insensitive, minor debridement can be carried out at the bedside. However, in many cases the patient must be taken to the operating room for the adequate debridement under anesthesia. Taylor and Porter have demonstrated that aggressive foot debridement, and, when indicated, revascularization resulted in long term salvage of 73% of threatened limbs even in high risk patients [26]. Biopsy should be considered when the ulcer appears at an atypical location, e.g., not over the metatarsal heads or the plantar surface of the hallux, when it cannot be explained by trauma, and when it is unresponsive to aggressive therapy. On numerous occasions biopsies of atypical ulcers have revealed malignancies, both primary and metastatic.

Infection is a common and major complication of diabetic foot wounds. Infection leads to microthrombi formation, causing further ischaemia, necrosis, and progressive gangrene. Massive infection is the most common factor leading to amputation. Lichter et al. reviewed the laboratory results of a large series of patients with serious pedal infection [27]. In this series the sedimentation rates were significantly elevated, mean 58.6 mm/h. Surprisingly, the mean white count was only 9,700. Therefore, one should not depend on white counts alone as a measure of the seriousness of the foot infection. As with other series, they found the lesions to be polymicrobial, 72% having gram positive cocci and 49% gram negative. Nine percent had gram negative anaerobes [27]. There is a high correlation between foot ulcers, infection and other diabetic complications.

Lichter et al. found that 67% of these patients had retinopathy, 70% nephropathy, 80% peripheral neuropathy, 91% decreased peripheral pulses, 69% hypertension and 40% atherosclerotic heart disease [27]. The selection of an oral antibiotic or parenteral antibiotic for the treatment of a diabetic foot infection is based on medical judgment. It should be kept in mind that many diabetic foot infections contain gram negative organisms. Therefore the oral antibiotic chosen should be effective for gram positive and gram negative organisms. The criterion for hospitalization and treatment with parenteral antibiotics includes patients who are septic, febrile, and have leukocytosis and deep infection. The patient with what appears to be a minor infection on the plantar surface of the foot and evidence of infection on the dorsum of the foot, suggested by erythema and frequently oedema, should be hospitalized. Even though the patient is not septic, there is high probability that severe infection exists deep in the foot. Patients with infection and severe PAD and infection should be hospitalized and evaluated for arterial by-pass surgery. The worst scenario leading to amputation is ischaemia and infection. Patients with PAD should be given parenteral antibiotics to achieve higher concentration of antibiotics in the peripheral tissues that cannot be achieved by oral therapy alone. Furthermore, the antibiotic of choice frequently can only be given parenterally. If an oral antibiotic is selected, patient should be examined regularly [22]. Infection in the diabetic can deteriorate rapidly within twenty-four hours. It is therefore our recommendation that diabetics on oral therapy should be seen within a few days following institution of therapy. They must be carefully instructed to notify the physician at once should there be an increase in redness, drainage, pain, odour, or evidence of lymphangitis. While many of these patients have insensate feet, the development of pain is indicative of deep infection and requires immediate attention. The development of a bad odour also indicates worsening infection and frequently the presence of anaerobes. It is very important that in patients with infection their blood sugar level must be monitored closely. A rising blood sugar level strongly suggests worsening infection, even though other signs and symptoms of a worsening infection are absent. When infection is not responding to aggressive debridement and antibiotic therapy, the wound should be debrided again and recultured, as the flora may have changed. Chronic recurrent or resistant infection suggests the presence of osteomyelitis. Impending or developing gangrene also suggests possible progression of infection. Indications of worsening infection are noted in Table 2.

Table 2 [25]

Table 2
Worsening infection: Indications

Signs and Symptoms
Increased:
  Drainage
  Erythema
  Pain
  Temperature
  Malodorous
  Lymphangitis
  Lymphadenopathy
  Gangrene
Laboratory
Increased:
  Blood Sugar
  WBC
  Sedimentation Rate

Osteomyelitis is a frequent complication of diabetic foot ulcers and infection. Osteomyelitis may be difficult to detect on a clinical basis. Newman and coworkers showed that in biopsy-proven osteomyelitis only one third of the patients had clinically suspected osteomyelitis [28]. If bone is visible or the ulcer can be probed to bone, the probability of the presence of osteomyelitis is extremely strong. Scanning techniques for osteomyelitis are not always successful. The triple phase scan with technetium lacks specificity[29]. Magnetic-resonance imaging (MRI) is proving to be a helpful technique. However, Newman and coworkers[30] found the use of labeled-leukocyte Indium $_{111}$ scanning techniques to be superior to magnetic resonance imaging[30].

Bamberger, Daus, and Gerding established prognostic factors for preventing amputation in the face of osteomyelitis[31]. They found that in patients without necrosis, gangrene, or the presence of swelling, the use of antimicrobial therapy active against the isolated pathogens given intravenously for at least four weeks of combined intravenously and orally for 10 weeks predicted a good outcome without the need for ablative surgical procedures[31]. Lipsky et al have recently reviewed soft tissue and bone infection in the diabetic foot[32]. Metabolic control is essential. It has been well demonstrated in a number of studies that leukocyte function is impaired in the presence of uncontrolled diabetes. Blood sugar levels should be kept below 200 mg/dl and as close to euglycaemia as is reasonable. Soaking the feet has no benefit, although it has been traditional approach. Soaking can lead to maceration and further infection. Because of the insensitive foot, soaking may take place in water that is too hot, resulting in severe burns. Chemical soaks can result in chemical burns[33]. Oedema is frequently present. Elevation of the feet, no more than the thickness of one pillow, can be beneficial. Higher elevation may impede circulation. Avoidance of weight bearing is essential. These patients have insensitive feet and because the ulcer is not painful, they continue to walk. The result is an increase in pressure necrosis, forcing bacteria deeper into the tissues, and causing failure to heal. The use of crutches and wheelchairs is seldom successful in achieving total and consistent avoidance of weight bearing.

Many patients with PN have ataxia, making the use of crutches potentially dangerous. The best method for avoidance of weight bearing in appropriately selected patients is the use of the contact cast. The contact cast allows the patient to be ambulatory but essentially avoids weight bearing by redistributing the weight and decreasing the pressure on the ulcerated area[34, 35]. When an ulcer does not heal despite good metabolic control, adequate debridement, parenteral antibiotic therapy and avoidance of weight bearing, the impaired healing may be caused by vascular insufficiency. Mills, et al, found that all appropriately treated neuropathic ulcers and forefoot infections healed in-patients with palpable pedal pulses. If foot pulses were absent and arteriography confirmed large-vessel occlusive disease, foot lesions and infections healed when concomitant revascularization was done[36].

The worst scenario for impaired would healing or the clearing of infection may be vascular insufficiency. Ankle brachial indexes of less than 0.45 or transcutaneous oxygen pressure<30 mm Hg and certainly those under 20mm Hg are highly predictive that the infection will not resolve and that the ulcer will not heal. For example, Pecoraro and colleagues found a 39-fold increased risk of early wound failure if the average peri-wound transcutaneous oxygen pressure was less than 22 mm Hg[34]. Vascular surgery should always be considered in these cases. The importance of peripheral arterial reconstruction was demonstrated by LoGerfo and associates. IN 2883 extreme distal arterial reconstructions, they found a statistically significant decrease in every category of amputation, a decrease that correlated precisely with increasing the rate of dorsalis pedis artery by-pass[37]. Hyperbaric oxygen delivered by the hyperbaric chamber has been reported to be helpful in healing diabetic foot ulcers [38]. Hyperbaric oxygen delivered by hyperbaric boot is totally ineffective. It must be kept in mind that the hyperbaric oxygen is used in conjunction with all of the aggressive treatments outlined in Table 1. Experimental studies have suggested that a combination of topical growth factors and hyperbaric oxygen maybe beneficial in improving wound healing[39].

TOPICAL TREATMENT OF FOOT ULCERS.

The use of topical therapy goes back to ancient times, when an unbelievable number of substances were used to treat wounds, ranging from wine to human excreta (Table-Talk, XCII "Of Good's Works," Martin Luther 1483-1546). Today the list of topical agents remains long and continues to grow. Currently resins and enzyme therapy to aid in debridement are advocated by some. Although these are of some benefit, they represent adjunct therapy and should not be substituted for aggressive surgical debridement. It has been traditional to use povidone-iodine (Betadine) acetic acid, hydrogen peroxide, and sodium hypochlorite (Dakin's solution). Although these substances destroy surface bacteria, they are cytotoxic to granulation tissue and may delay would healing[40]. It is therefore ideally, that these substances should be either avoided or used for the shortest periods. The benefits of topically applied antibacterial agents, silver sulfadiazine (1%), polymixin B with bacitracin and neomycin, and gentamicin sulfate may be helpful[40]. Topical antibiotics alone may not be satisfactory, and the use of oral or parenteral antibiotics in conjunction with topical therapy is frequently necessary. Cleansing agent and types of dressings can make a difference in the rate of wound healing. Moist dressings seem to aid wound healing[40]. Despite aggressive therapy and adequate circulation, some diabetic foot ulcers heal slowly or not at all. Current investigative studies with topically applied platelet-derived growth factors to these foot ulcers have shown these factors to be important adjunct therapy in would healibng[41,42].

Bentkover and Champion have shown the cost effectiveness of would care centers and the use of platelet releasate[43]. Platelet-derived would healing formula is an autologous solution extracted from the alpha granules of the patient's platelets. This extract is applied to the ulcer daily by the patient in an outpatient setting. The platelet-derived wound healing formula contains several growth factors. They are platelet-derived growth factor, angiogenesis factor, epidermal factor, transforming growth factor B, and platelet factor 4. Recent work has shown that interactions between factors and the extracellular matrix are of central importance in the process that causes wounds to close. Transforming growth factor B appears to be a central player in many of the steps of wound healing, inducing angiogenesis, acting as a chemo attractant for macrophages and fibroblasts, regulating self proliferation, and stimulating extracellular matrix[44]. The impediments to wound healing are listed in Table 3.

TABLE 3 [25]: IMPEDIMENTS TO WOUND HEALING

1. Vascular

a. Atherosclerosis

b. Increased viscosity

2. Neurologic

a. Insensate foot

b. Decreased flare reaction

3. Infection

a) Inadequate debridement
b) Poor vascularity
c) Microthrombi
d) Hyperglycemia
e) Decreased polymorpho nuclear leucocyte function
f) Polymicrobial infection
g) Changing bacteria
h) Osteomyelitis

4. Immunosuppression

5. Mechanical

a. Oedema

b. Weight bearing

6. Poor nutrition

a. Low serum albumin level

7. Decreased growth factors

8. Poor patient compliance

9. Delayed treatment and referral

POST-TREATMENT MANAGEMENT OF HEALED DIABETIC FOOT ULCER:

Foot Ulcers:

Even though the diabetic foot ulcer has healed, the job is not complete. The underlying aetiologies responsible for the ulcer, such as foot deformity, calluses, and increased pressure are still present. In addition, scar tissue from previously healed ulcers is not strong tissue and is thus vulnerable to the shearing forces of walking. Special measures are therefore necessary protect the vulnerable sites of previous ulceration. These include education of the patient in walking, for example, taking shorter steps and decreasing overall walking. Patients whose jobs require standing or walking, such as waiters or waitresses, may need to change jobs. Therapeutic footwear plays a very important role in preventing recurrence of these ulcers.

Special Footwear:

The use of special therapeutic footwear is critical in preventing ulceration or recurrence. Patients who have cocked-up toes require a shoe with a bigger toe box. The patient with a markedly deformed foot, such as the Charcot foot, need a specially molded shoe. An in-depth shoe with a plastic-like material, such as plastazote insole, is frequently required to redistribute the weight away from the previously ulcerated site and thus prevent recurrence of ulcer. The importance of special shoes was clearly demonstrated at a study at King's College in London, which showed an 83% recurrence of ulcers when patients returned to wearing regular shores; with the use of special shoes, there was only a 17% recurrence of ulceration [45].

Off-loading:

Increased plantar pressure is one of the main cause for ulceration in the diabetic population. Healing of these ulcers requires adequate blood supply, control of infection, excellent wound care and 'offloading' or pressure redistribution of the ulcerative area. Of all these factors, 'offloading' is a unique challenge in treating chronic wounds.

Diabetic foot ulcer is a complex pathological process with a narrow window of opportunity to work with. If not dealt with right approach it unfortunately ends up in amputation. Hence it requires special care.

A non-healing ulcer on plantar aspect can cause spread of infection. Eighty percent of diabetic foots are neuropathic in India. This leads to loss of sensation in foot and offloading is the most important solution for healing of plantar lesions.

Some of the offloading techniques that have been used are:

1. Total contact cast (TCC)

2. Walker

3. Air cast shoe

4. Complete bed rest.

All the above mentioned techniques have several drawbacks and the most important being poor patient compliance and high cost.

An ideal off-loading device should be:

1. Patient compliant

2. Easy to apply

3. Cost effective

4. Does not require special training

5. Effective in healing the wound

6. Ambulation with device should be comfortable.

7. Should be accommodated in diabetic foot wear with ease.

8. Should be practiced at all levels of rural healthcare systems and by paramedical staff.

Keeping all of these guidelines in mind, a study was carried out in our institution by Dr. T. Arun, where a simple offloading device called "MANDAKINI", was used which cost less than INR 10 to make, didn't not require any special skills, was easily reproducible, had good patient compliance and produced very satisfactory results. This device was designed by Dr. Sunil V. Kari from Karnataka, India in 2009.[92]

Materials required to make the device was a pair of used gloves and a roll of elastocrepe plaster. The technique of making the device is illustrated in the picture below. The device could be reapplied daily and had to be changed only every 4 weeks.

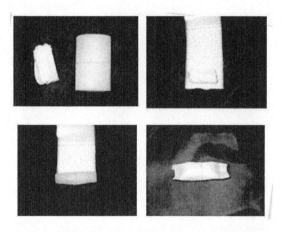

It was randomized control study and patients were randomized to two groups, one received this off-loading device and the other did not have any offloading. The patients were monitored daily by the same surgeon and the ulcer size and depth were recorded in all patients. All patients were treated with appropriate antibiotics, insulin and daily dressing. The patient progress was recorded at 2, 4, 6 weeks. They were also categorized based on the cross-sectional area of the ulcers. All groups were matched with cases and controls alike. The table below will demonstrate that off-loading with this simple and inexpensive device has led to faster ulcer healing compared to the controls.

RESULTS

ULCER HEALING IN 2 WEEKS (Table A)			
OFF LOADED		NO OFFLOADING	
Percentage healing	No of patients	Percentage healing	No of patients
<25%	0	<25%	17
25%	7	25%	8
50%	18	50%	0
75%	0	75%	0
100%	0	100%	0
Total	25	Total	25

ULCER HEALING IN 4 WEEKS (Table B)			
OFF LOADED		NO OFFLOADING	
Percentage healing	No of patients	Percentage healing	No of patients
<25%	0	<25%	0
25%	0	25%	17
50%	7	50%	5
75%	18	75%	3
100%	0	100%	0
Total	25	Total	25

ULCER HEALING IN 6 WEEKS (Table C)			
OFF LOADED		NO OFFLOADING	
Percentage healing	No of patients	Percentage healing	No of patients
<25%	0	<25%	0
25%	0	25%	3
50%	0	50%	2
75%	7	75%	13
100%	18	100%	7
Total	25	Total	25

Teamwork:

The management of the diabetic foot requires the interaction of many medical disciplines (The Table 4). A team approach is needed that will save the foot, not amputate it.

Table 4: Team members involved in the care of the diabetic foot [25]

1. Primary physician

2. Endocrinologist

3. Diabetologist

4. Podiatrist

5. Nurse educator

6. Physician's assistant

7. Enterostomal nurse

8. Infectious disease specialist

9. Neurologist

10. Vascular surgeon

11. Orthopedist

12. Physiatrist

13. Pedortrist

14. Orthotist

15. Physical therapist

16. Prosthetist

17. Occupational therapist

18. Social worker

19. Home care nurse

Patient Education:

Of all the approaches to prevent ulceration and to save the diabetic foot, the most important is patient education. Despite our current knowledge, physicians cannot totally prevent PAD and PN. However, the patients can be educated in proper foot care, and can learn how to prevent injury and detect lesions as early as possible. At the time of outpatient clinic visits and while the footwear is off, the nurse or physician should review the do's and don'ts of foot care with the patient. This objective cannot be adequately accomplished simply by handing the patients a list of instructions. The instruction should be explained and questions should be encouraged and answered, so that the patients can attain a better understanding of the importance of foot care (Table 5). These instructions should be carried out at least once a year or even more often. The effectiveness of educational program in reducing amputation has been noted by Malone and co-workers (46) and more recently by Litzelman[47].

Table 5 [25]

Patient-instructions for the care of the diabetic foot

1) Do not smoke.
2) Inspect the feet daily for blisters, cuts and scratches. The use of mirror can aid in seeing the bottom of the feet. Always check between the toes.
3) Wash feet daily, dry carefully, especially between the toes.

4) Avoid extremes of temperatures. Test water with hand, elbow or thermometer before bathing,

5) If feet feel cold at night, wear socks. Do not apply hot water bottles or heating pads. Do not use an electric blanket. Do not soak feet in hot water.

6) Do not walk on hot surfaces such as sandy beaches, or on cement around swimming pools.

7) Do not walk barefooted.

8) Do not use chemical agents for removal of corns and calluses, corn plasters or strong antiseptic solutions.

9) Do not use adhesive tape on the feet.

10) Inspect the insides of shoes daily for foreign objects, nail points, torn linings and rough areas.

11) If your vision is impaired, have a family member inspect feet daily, trim nails and buff calluses.

12) Do not soak feet.

13) For dry feet, use a very thin coat of lubricating oil or cream. Apply after bathing and drying the feet. Do not put oil or cream between the toes. Consult your physician for detailed instructions.

14) Wear properly fitting stockings. Do not wear mended stocking with seams. Change stockings daily.

15) Do not wear garters.

16) Footwear should be comfortable at time of purchase. Do not depend on them to stretch out.

Shoes should be made of leather. Purchase shoes late in the afternoon when feet are the largest. Running or special walking shoes may be worn after checking with your physician. Purchase shoes from a shoe salesperson who understands diabetic foot problems.

17) Do not wear shoes without stockings.

18) Do not wear sandals with thongs between the toes.

19) In winter, take special precautions. Wear wool socks and protective foot gear such as fleece lined boots.

20) Cut nails straight across.

21) Do not cut corns and calluses; follow instructions from your physician or podiatrist.

22) See your physician regularly and be sure that your feet are examined at each visit.

23) Notify your physician or podiatrist at once should you develop a blister or sore on your foot.

24) Be sure to inform your podiatrist that you are diabetic.

RISK FACTORS FOR LOWER EXTREMITY AMPUTATIONS

Diabetic foot ulcers more commonly proceed to amputation in male patients [48, 49]

Mehmood et al of Pakistan in his paper on clinical profile and management outcome of diabetic foot ulcers in a tertiary care hospital determined that out of 120 patients majority of patients who underwent amputation were type 2 diabetic patients (95.7%), males (66%), with duration of diabetes more than 10 years (p<0.05). The mean age was 54.29+/-7.71 years [48].

Al-Maskari et al studied the prevalence of risk factors for diabetic foot complications. Out of 513 diabetic patients (mean age of 53 years), 39% had peripheral neuropathy and 12% had peripheral vascular disease. Significant risk factors were male gender, poor level of education, increased duration of diabetes and presence of hypertension[49].

The duration of diabetes plays a very important role in amputation. Most studies reveal that the incidence of amputation increases more than 10 yrs of duration.

Krittiyawong et al revealed the prevalence and risk factors associated with lower extremity amputation in Thai diabetics. This cross sectional study revealed mean duration of diabetes was 10 years. Out of 556 patients 370 patients had peripheral vascular disease (PVD), 64.1% had toe amputations. Multiple logistic regression analysis of risk factors revealed a high risk of lower extremity amputation in peripheral vascular disease, diabetic retinopathy and in patients with ulcer[50].

Leelawattana et al in her project of prevalence of vascular complications in long standing type 2 diabetes described that the complications were amputation (5.5%), stroke (9.4), and foot ulcer (13.4%). The project involved 9284 patients of which 2244 were of long standing type 2 diabetics-mean duration 7.0+/-3.9 years[51].

Nephropathy, neuropathy and retinopathy are the most important factors which lead to lower extremity amputation in diabetic foot ulcer patients.

Miyajima et al studied the risk factors for major limb amputation in diabetic foot gangrene patients. One hundred and ten patients underwent amputation out of 210 patients with diabetic foot ulcer (DFU). 45 had major amputation and 65 had minor amputation. The blood glucose control was poor in all the major amputees with a mean

HbAlc (8.8). Nephropathy and arteriosclerosis were considered important to avoid major amputations[52].

Peter et al described the influence of physical, psychological and social factors in diabetic lower extremity amputation. History of previous amputation (P=0.01), peripheral vascular disease (p=0.007, OR = 5.5), peripheral neuropathy as measured with vibratory perception (OR 3.4, p=0.044) were the physical factors which were more significant than the psychological and social factors[53].

Margolis et al compared the association between renal failure and foot ulcer or lower extremity amputation in patients with diabetes. The study proved that there is a strong association between chronic kidney disease and diabetic foot ulcer irrespective of the presence or absence of peripheral disease, Patients even with moderate chronic kidney disease(<60ml/min per $1.73m^2$) had an increased risk of diabetic foot ulcer or lower extremity amputation[54].

Alder et al discovered the independent effects of PVD, sensory neuropathy and foot ulcer in diabetic patients with lower extremity amputation. His study revealed that peripheral sensory neuropathy, PVD foot ulcers, former amputation were independent risk factors for LEA[55]

The Wisconsin epidemiologic study of diabetic retinopathy of 14 year incidence of lower extremity amputation in diabetic patients by Moss et al concluded high blood pressure, history or ulcers, more severe retinopathy, high glycosylated Haemoglobin were significant risk factors for LEA[56]

Al-Tawfiq from Saudi Arabia evaluated the presentation and outcome of diabetic foot ulcers in Saudi Arabian patients. Out of 62 patients (mean age 64.8 years) all patients with diabetic foot ulcers of Wagner grade 4 or 5, hypertension, PVD, absence of pedal pulses and ischemic heart disease underwent amputation[57]

Elliot et al analyzed that large fiber dysfunction in diabetic peripheral neuropathy is predicted by cardiovascular risk factors. Large fibre dysfunction as measured by vibration perception threshold predicts foot ulceration, amputation and mortality. Vibration perception threshold (VPT) was measured by biothesiometry on 1407 patients with mean duration diabetes 14.7 +/-9.3 years mean age of 32.7+/-10.2 years. The result was abnormal VPT had increased the incidence of amputation. VPT was influenced by duration of diabetes, high HbAlc, male sex ($p=0.01$), diabetic retinopathy and nephropathy ($p=0.001$)[58].

In 2007, Casellini et al from USA published the clinical manifestations and current treatment options for diabetic neuropathies. The final outcome distal symmetric poly neuropathy the most common form of diabetic neuropathy usually involves small and large nerve fibers. Small nerve fiber neuropathy often presents with pain and loss of intraepidermal nerve fibres, but without objective signs or electrophysiological evidence of nerve damage. This type of neuropathy is a component of impaired glucose tolerance and the metabolic syndrome. The greatest risk from small fiber neuropathy is foot ulceration, subsequent gangrene and amputation. Large fiber neuropathy produces ataxia, incoordination, thus impairing activities of daily living causing falls and fractures. Duloxetine hydrochloride and Pregabalin have been approved for the treatment of neuropathic pain[59]

Vishwanathan et al had elaborated that the prevalence of infection was 6-11% amputation 3% in a study group of 1319. Neuropathy was significant factor leading to amputation (15%)[60].

A case control study of the risk factors for toe amputation in a diabetic population by Carlson et al shows obvious risk factors for toe amputation were male sex, osteomyelitis, digital deformity, diabetic nephropathy, neuropathy, and ischemia[61].

Amputation in diabetic patients Van Damme et al suggests end stage renal failure as a risk for amputation[62]

Explanations for the high risk of diabetes-related amputation in Caribbean population of Blank African decent and potential for prevention by Hennis et al from Barbados confirmed that PVD, peripheral neuropathy, high HbAlc, poor foot wear was the cause of increased amputation.[63].

Moss et al in the cohort study of Retinal Vascular changes and 20 year incidence of Lower extremity amputation has concluded that focal retinal arteriolar narrowing may reflect damage to the microvasculature, which itself manifests elsewhere in the body as a need for LEA[64.]

Alwaked et al studied concomitant macro and microvascular complication in diabetic nephropathy. Out of 1952 type 2 diabetic patients the mean age was 66.9+/-11.4 years, mean duration of diabetes was 15.4+/-7.5 years the mean age of onset of nephropathy was 61.5+/- 12.4 years, mean duration of nephropathy was 3.9+/-3.8 years. The complications were limb amputation (3.7%) retinopathy (11.7%), peripheral neuropathy (24.9%), myocardial infarction (24.1%), and acute coronary syndrome

(36.1%). The relative risks of developing these complications were significant after the onset nephropathy[65.]

A fourfold increase in foot ulcers in type 2 diabetic subjects without an increase in major amputation by a multidisciplinary setting was a review from Denmark by Hedetoft et al. The end result was neuropathy and ischemia were important risk factors for amputation $(p<0.05)$[66]

The article of Infection and diabetic foot by Senneville et al found that the consequence of a pre-existing foot wound whose chronicity is facilitated by the factors such as neuropathy and PVD, which is a factor of poor outcome, especially regarding the risk for leg amputation[67].

A study of 217 patients from university of Malaya Medical centre to evaluate the pre valence and risk factors for diabetic retinopathy by Tajunisah et al were duration of diabetes, hypertension, and presence of systemic complications (diabetic foot ulcer, lower limb amputation, nephropathy and peripheral neuropathy). The association of lower limb amputation and diabetic retinopathy was stressed n this study[68]

Risk of amputation in patients with diabetic foot ulcers: a claims – based study by Markowitz et al stated amputation to be high in males (AOR 1.98) Charlson comorbidity score of 4-5 and 6+ S (AOR=2.89) renal disease (AOR=2.11), PVD (AOR = 2.67), The study was on 5911 patients who showed an amputation rate of 2.3 amputation per 100 person years[69].

Reducing the incidence of foot ulceration and amputation in diabetes by Bartus et al states the incidence of foot ulcers range from (1.0%-4.1%). Amputation risk ranges from 2.1% to 13.7% per 1000. The common risk factors include neuropathy, retinopathy and PVD and trauma[70].

The risk factors for amputation are increased Wagner's grade and presence of comorbidities which are frequently hypertension, hyperlipidemia and ischemic heart disease.

Dos Santos et al from Brazil in 2006 identified the risk factors for primary major amputation in diabetic patients. Out of 99 patients the variables that favored amputations was male sex, sixth decade of life, type 2 diabetes, chronic arterial insufficiency, duration of diabetes, Wagner's classification. The important major amputation included age, ascending lymphangitis (OR 2.5), and Wagner grade (OR 3.4), and chronic arterial insufficiency without revascularization (OR 5.4) [71].

Frequency of lower extremity amputation in diabetics with reference to diabetic control and Wagner grades by Imran et al of Pakistan observed 60 patients of various Wagner grades 0-5 and showed that the frequency of major amputation increases with higher Wagner grades and poor glycemic control. (21.42%) in grade III (55.55%) in grade IV and (100%) in grade V had major amputation. In minor amputation 16.6% in grade I, (23.7%) in grade II, (57.14%) in grade III (44.44%), in grade IV underwent the amputation[72].

ISCHEMIA AND NEED FOR RE-VASCULARISATION IN LOWER EXTREMITY AMPUTATION.

Dalla et al in his study on treatment of diabetic foot ulcer: an overview strategies for clinical approach proved PVD is the main risk factor for amputation. PVD is not only in distal pulses but fully involves femoral, popliteal, tibial pulses. It can be treated with open or endovascular surgical procedures. Also Charcot's neuroarthropathy is a particular complication of neuropathy which leads to fragmentation and destruction of bones and joints[73].

Davis et al in the Fremantle diabetes study of predictors, consequences and costs of diabetes- related lower extremity amputation complicating diabetes interpreted ABPI < 0.9, high HbAlc, neuropathy were the risk factors for LEA[74].

Epidemiology of diabetes foot problems and predictive factors for limb loss by Nather et al from Singapore. This prospective study on 202 patients had significant univariate predictive factors for limb loss were age above 60 years, stroke, IHD, nephropathy, retinopathy, PVD, ABPI<0.8, gangrene, infection and MRSA. Upon multiple logistic regression PVD and infection were significant factors for LEA[75].

Diabetic foot ulcers revascularization when feasible and improve blood flow and hasten wound healing. Amputation is also prevented by proper education of diabetic patients, foot care and appropriate foot wear. This was proved by Unnikrishan et al in his paper an "Approach to the diabetic foot"[76].

Faglia et al in his prospective study of peripheral angioplasty (PTA) as the first choice revascularization procedure in diabetic patients with critical limb ischemia evaluated 993 patients who underwent peripheral angioplasty. The 5 year primary patency was 88%. He has proved that PTA as the first choice revascularization procedure is feasible, safe and effective for limb salvage in a high percentage of diabetic patients. Clinical re-stenosis was an infrequent event and PTA could successfully be repeated in most cases[77]

Wijeyaratnae et al in his publication in 2003,"revascularization in diabetic small vessel disease of lower limbs: Is it worthwhile?", used saphenous vein to bypass occluded infra popliteal arteries in diabetics with critical leg ischemia over a 5- year period on 23 patients, He noted patency in 65% of patents at a mean follow up of 3 months. He concluded that bypass of diabetic small vessel disease of the lower limbs is feasible and effective in preventing major amputation and maintaining independent mobility[78].

In 1996 De Campo et al from Canada in his case report on Microvascular free myocutaneous flap for treatment of non healing ischemic ulcers of the lower extremity. He discovered that arterial reconstruction alone has failed to stimulate healing of lesions with exposed bone and tendons in weight –bearing areas. But with a combination of percutaneous trans luminal angioplasty and a microvascular free myocutaneous flap, complete healing of the ulcer was noted and flap was visible for 35 months[79]

Lavery et al proved the four consistent dominant clusters for diabetic foot ulcers and amputation were 1) neuropathy, deformity, callus and elevated peak pressure, 2) PVD, 3) penetrating trauma, 4) ill fitting shoes. These four factors if prevented interrupt the cascade of events that lead to amputation [80]

Risk factors associated with adverse outcomes in a population based prospective cohort study of people with their first diabetic foot ulcer by Winkly et al of UK explained the variable were age, male gender, smoking , ulcer site, size, severity of neuropathy, ischemia, HbAlc levels, presence of vascular complication. In a group of 253 patients 36 patients had amputations (15.5%) microvascular complications were the only explanation for recurrent ulceration[81]

Risk assessment of the diabetic foot and wound by Wu et al in 2005 stated the key factor associated with the non healing of diabetic foot wound and therefore amputation include wound depth, presence of infection and presence of ischemia[82]

"Diabetic heel ulcers: major risk factors for lower extremity amputation (LEA)", by Younes et al describes out of all foot ulcers seen in diabetic patients heel ulcers are the most serious and often lead to LEA. The most common risk factors for ulceration in the heel is immobility of the lower limbs, retinopathy, PVD, structural deformity, and poor foot hygiene[83]

Frykberg et al in his study of diabetic foot ulcers: pathogenesis and management in 2002 proved the most frequent etiologies are neuropathy, trauma, deformity, PVD and high plantar pressures. A multidisciplinary management is needed that focuses on prevention, patient education, regular foot examination optimal use of therapeutic foot wear has reduced the incidence of LEA[84].

Chaturvedi et al in his article of risk of diabetes – related amputation in south Asians vs. Europeans in the UK, observed a decrease by quarter in the risk of amputation in south Asians as compared with Europeans. This was explained by low rates of PVD, neuropathy and smoking in south Asians as compared with the Europeans[85]

AIMS AND OBJECTIVES

- To identify the risk factors in diabetic patients contributing to the persistent, non-healing, and progression of foot ulcer requiring amputation of the lower extremity.

MATERIALS AND METHODS

STUDY DESIGN

This was a prospective study on a group of 120 patents who were already diagnosed diabetic patients with foot ulcer. The study period was from August 2007 to July 2009. The risk factors contributing to lower extremity amputation in patients with diabetic foot ulcers were identified from 53 patients who underwent amputation of 120 patients involved in this study. The approval from the ethics committee of Mahatma Gandhi Medical College & Research Institute was obtained for performing this study.

STUDY POPULATION

All diabetic patients with foot ulcer and gangrene of toes and foot presenting to the surgical outpatient department of Mahatma Gandhi Medical College hospital were recruited in this study after obtaining informed consent.

INCLUSION CRITERIA

All known diabetic patient with foot ulcers presenting to the surgical outpatient department of Mahatma Gandhi medical college hospital were included, after obtaining their informed consent.

EXCLUSION CRITERIA

Patients with foot ulcers in non diabetic patients and ulcer due to other causes (eg: Trauma, malignancy)

METHODOLOGY

An informed consent was obtained from each patient before recruitment to this study, after fully explaining the nature of study and the possible investigations involved in this study.

On admission a thorough clinical history was obtained regarding the mode of onset of ulcer, its progression, duration and type of diabetes, type of medications, use of regular footwear, associated comorbidities as hypertension, hyperlipidemia, risk factors of smoking and alcohol consumption.

Then a thorough clinical examination was carried out including general examination, detailed examination of the affected foot, regarding the size of the ulcer, site of ulcer, pus discharge, deformity of toes, viability of toes, presence of peripheral pulses in the leg (posterior tibial & dorsalis pedis), presence of touch and vibration – Then ophthalmology opinion was obtained on all the patients regarding the presence of retinopathy.

All routine blood investigation such as full blood count, blood urea, serum creatinine, serum electrolytes, random blood sugar, and serum albumin, urine for routine examination, micro albuminuria and radiograph of the affected foot was obtained on admission. The following day lipid profile, fasting and post-prandial blood sugar value was measured.

On admission pus for culture and sensitivity was done and antibiotics started accordingly. All the slough and necrotic material was debrided in the bedside and daily dressings with antiseptic solution was done.

All patients were assessed on daily basis for their general condition, control of blood sugar and appropriate control of blood sugar was achieved based on the opinion by the Diabetologist of Mahatma Gandhi medical college. The ulcers were inspected on daily basis. Surgical debridement was done to remove the slough and necrotic material whenever necessary.

Patients who had signs of ascending infection not controlled with antibiotics and debridement, gangrene, osteomyelitis, exposed tendons and joints had amputation above the site of the infection. Patients who had signs of toxemia underwent major amputation.

PROCEDURE

The current status of the limb, ulcer and the need for amputation including the benefits and complications of the procedure was completely informed to the patient and their attenders in their own language. A written informed consent was obtained before performing the procedure.

Minor amputation was done by infiltrating local anesthesia 2% Lignocaine in the surrounding area and the affected toe was removed till fresh bleeding and viable tissue is seen. The exposed bone or the head of the metatarsals was nibbled to expose the bone marrow to facilitate wound healing.

Patient requiring major amputation were taken up for surgery under spinal anaesthesia. Below knee or above knee amputation were performed depending on the level of infection. The wound was left open or primarily closed depending on the level of infection. All patients were monitored regularly, the wound site was inspected daily and daily dressings were done. Stringent control of blood sugar was obtained in liaison with the Diabetologist including treatment and dietary pattern. Patients who underwent major amputation were motivated for the use of prosthesis and rehabilitation was organized in liaison with the Physiotherapist.

FOLLOW UP

All patients were reviewed after discharge in the surgical outpatient department once in every 2 weeks for 3 times consecutively, then as required subsequently.

END POINT

Healing of the ulcer or amputation was considered as the end point of the study.

Healing was defined as complete healing of the raw area and formation of good scar tissue.

Partial healing defined as good granulation tissue without slough or necrotic material.

STASTISTICAL METHODS

Out of the 53 patients who underwent amputation, univariate analysis, multivariate logistic regression (Wald' test), was done on the risk factors which included smoking, consumption of alcohol, site of the ulcer, duration of diabetes, gender predisposition, presence of peripheral pulses, ankle brachial pressure index, associated complications such as neuropathy, nephropathy and retinopathy. P value of less than 0.05 was considered significant.

OBSERVATIONS & RESULTS

This study was a prospective study to identify the risk factors leading to lower extremity amputation, in known diabetic patients presenting with foot ulcers. This study was carried out in Mahatma Gandhi Medical College & Research Institute, from a period of August 2007 to July 2009. One hundred and twenty known diabetic patients with foot ulcers were studied after obtaining informed written consent.

The age of the patients ranged from 32 to 78 years with a peak incidence of presentation in the 5th decade of life. Forty four patients (36.37%) were in the age group of 41-50 years of age followed by 30 patients (25.0%) in the 6th decade of life. The incidence is (18.3%) in the 3rd decade, (15.8) in the 7th decade and (4.1%) in the 8th decade of life as stated in (Table 1 & Figure 1)

The incidence of foot ulcer is increases with the increase in the duration of diabetes. Out of the 120 patients who presented with foot ulcers, 78 patients (65%) had diabetes more than 5 years (Table 2 & Figure 2). Table 2 also describes the number of patients with their duration of diabetes.

Thirty eight male patients (71.7%) underwent amputation out of 53 patients which signifies that males are more prone for amputation as shown in (Table 3 & Figure 3).

Out of 120 patients (75.8%) of the patients were on Insulin and oral hypoglycemic agents while (24.2%) were exclusively on oral hypoglycemic agents for their control of blood sugar (Table 4)

Table 5 shows the relation between the risk factors namely smoking (52.5%) and alcohol consumption (45%) and the incidence of foot ulcers. Hypertension (71.7%) and hyperlipidemia (81.7%) were significant comorbidities that led to the development of foot ulcers (Table 5).

The presence of distal pulses in the whole group of 120 patients is described in Table 6. Posterior tibial was present in (82.5%) and dorsalis pedis was present in (68.3%). The pulses were evaluated by clinical and hand Doppler (Table 6).

The site of ulcer was mostly in the fore foot region (72.5%) followed by mid foot ulcers (20%) and hind foot ulcer (7.5%) as shown in (Table 7 & Figure 4).

The microorganisms which grew on microbiology culture and sensitivity were predominantly Proteus (26.7%), followed by E.coli (20.8%), polymicrobial (19.2%) respectively. Pseudomonas & klebsiella were (11.7%). Alpha hemolytic streptococci was (7.5%) and MRSA was the least which was (2.4%) (Table8).

Eleven patients (20.7%) had below knee amputation and 1 patient (2.0%) had above knee amputation. Minor amputation which was removal of toes was in 41 patients (77.3%) (Table9 & Figure 5).

The ankle brachial index in the amputated and non amputated group is compared in table 10. Only 23 out of 120 patients had normal Ankle Brachial index (ABPI) of 0.9 & above. Rest of the 97 patients had ABPI less than 0.9. Out of the 53 patients in the amputated group only 2 patients had ABPI of 0.9 and above (Table 10 & Figure 6).

Fifty percent of patient who underwent major amputation consumed alcohol and (58.3%) patients were smokers. In the minor amputation group (73.1%) were smokers and (65.8%) consumed alcohol and these factors are significant which led to amputation (Table 11 & Figure 7, 8).

The duration of diabetes plays an important role in amputation. 66.6% patients of major amputation and 87.8% patients of the minor amputation group had diabetes for more than 5 years (Table 12 & Figure 9).

Table 13 shows the site of ulcer in the foot of amputated patients. Out of the 12 major amputations 6 patients (50%) had fore foot ulcers. 4 patients (33.3%) had mid foot ulcers and 2 patients (16.7%) had hind foot ulcers.

The associated complications in 53 amputated patients were neuropathy (62.3%), retinopathy (62.3%) and nephropathy (49.1%) respectively as shown in (Table 14). They were not found to be statistically significant for amputation.

The peripheral pulses, posterior tibial and dorsalis pedis was present predominantly in most of amputated patients. Posterior tibial was present in (83%) and dorsalis pedis was present in (68%). In the major amputation group (58.3%) of patients had posterior tibial and (33.3%) dorsalis pedis pulsations detected either by clinical of hand Doppler. Similarly in the minor amputation group (90.2%) had posterior tibial and (78.0%) dorsalis pedis pulsation (Table 15).

Table 16 shows the univariate analysis of risk factors for amputation. Smoking and alcohol consumption was significant with a P value of 0.0014. P values for neuropathy, nephropathy, osteomyelitis and retinopathy were indeterminate. The P value for duration of diabetes longer than 5 years was 0.00049 and was significant. Male gender was also a significant risk factor with P value of 0.0301 along with peripheral vascular disease as measured by ABPI of less than 0.9 (P value=0.00035)

The risk factors had significant p values on univariate analysis when amputation group was compared with the non amputation group. But there was no statistical significance when univariate analysis was done on each factor when major and minor amputation groups were compared.

Upon multiple logistic regression (Wald's test) the only significant factors were male gender and ABPI of less than 0.9.

TABLE 1 : AGE AND SEX DISTRIBUTION OF PATIENTS WITH DIABETIC FOOT ULCERS						
Age	Male	%	Female	%	Total No. of Patients	Total %
31-40	10	8.3	12	10.0	22	18.3
41-50	32	26.7	12	10.0	44	36.7
51-60	14	11.6	16	13.3	30	25.0
61-70	13	10.8	6	5.0	19	15.8
71-80	4	3.4	1	0.8	5	4.2
Total	73	60.8	47	39.2	120	100

TABLE 2: DURATION OF DIABETES MELLITUS IN YEARS		
Duration of DM (in years)	No. of Patients	Percentage
<2	10	8.3
>2-3	11	9.2
>3-4	8	6.7
>4-5	13	10.8
>5-6	9	7.5
>6-7	10	8.3
>7-8	9	7.5
>8-9	17	14.1
>9-10	15	12.5
>10	18	15.1
Total	120	100

TABLE 3: GENDER AND AMPUTATION				
Gender	Amputation (n=53)		Non Amputation (n=67)	
	No.of Patients	%	No. of Patients	%
Male	38	71.7	35	52.3
Female	15	28.3	32	47.7
Total	53	100	67	100

TABLE 4: TYPE OF MEDICATIONS		
Medications	No. of Patients	Percentage
OHA only	29	24.2
Insulin+OHA	91	75.8
Total	120	100

TABLE 5: RISK FACTORS FOR FOOT ULCERS IN DIABETICS						
	Yes	Percentage	No.	Percentage	P value	Statistical significance
Smoking	63	52.5%	57	47.5%	0.4386	NO
Alcohol	54	45%	66	55%	0.1213	NO
Hypertension	86	71.7%	34	28.3%	**0.0000**	**SIGNIFICANT**
Hyperlipidemia	98	81.7%	22	18.3%	**0.0000**	**SIGNIFICANT**

TABLE 6: PERIPHERAL PULSES IN PATIENTS WITH DIABETIC FOOT ULCERS				
Peripheral Pulses	**Posterior Tibial**	**%**	**Dorsalis Pedis**	**%**
Present	99	82.5	82	68.3
Absent	21	17.5	38	31.7
Total	**120**	**100**	**120**	**100**

TABLE 7: SITE OF ULCER		
Site of Ulcer	No. of Patients	Percentage
Fore Foot	87	72.5
Mid Foot	24	20
Hind Foot	9	7.5
Total	120	100

TABLE 8: PUS CULTURE		
Microorganism	No. of Patients	Percentage
Proteus	32	26.7
E.coli	25	20.8
Pseudomonas	14	11.7
Klebsiella	14	11.7
Alpha hemolytic Streptococci	9	7.5
MRSA	3	2.4
Mixed growth	23	19.2
Total	120	100

TABLE 9: TYPE OF AMPUTATION CARRIED OUT IN PATIENTS WITH FOOT ULCERS		
Amputation	No. of Patients	Percentage
Below Knee	11	20.7
Above Knee	1	2.0
Toes	41	77.3
Total	53	100

TABLE 10: ANKLE BRACHIAL PRESSURE INDEX & AMPUTATION		
ABPI	No.(%)	AMPUTATION No. (%)
0.3-0.5	2(1.7)	2(100.0)
0.6	16(13.3)	16(100.0)
0.7	30(25.0)	15(50.0)
0.8	49(40.8)	18(36.7)
>0.9	23(19.2)	2(8.7)
TOTAL	120(100)	53(100)

*ABPI-clinical and hand Doppler.

TABLE 11: SMOKING AND ALCOHOL CONSUMPTION & AMPUTATION					
AMPUTATION	NO. OF PATIENTS OUT OF 53	SMOKING	%	ALCOHOL	%
MAJOR	12	7	58.3	6	50.0
MINOR	41	30	73.1	27	65.8
Total	53	37	69.8	33	62.3

TABLE 12: DURATION OF DIABETES MELLITUS AND AMPUTATION			
DURATION (years)	MAJOR AMPUTATION No. (%)	MINOR AMPUTATION No.(%)	TOTAL No.(%)
<5 years	4(33.4)	5(12.2)	9(16.8)
>5 years	8(66.6)	36(87.8)	44(83.2)
TOTAL	12(100)	41(100)	53(100)

TABLE 13: SITE OF ULCER IN AMPUTATED PATIENTS				
Amputation	Fore Foot	Mid Foot	Hind Foot	Total
MAJOR (n=12)	6	4	2	**12**
MINOR (n=41)	41	0	0	**41**

TABLE 14: ASSOCIATED COMPLICATIONS AND AMPUTATION						
COMPLICATION	MAJOR AMPUTATION (n=12)		MINOR AMPUTATION (n=41)		P value	STATISTICAL SIGNIFICANCE
	No. Of patients	%	No. Of patients	%		
NEUROPATHY	9	75.0	24	58.5	**0.3007**	NO
NEPHROPATHY	6	50.0	20	48.7	**0.9408**	NO
RETINOPATHY	8	66.6	25	60.9	**0.7206**	NO

TABLE 15: PERIPHERAL PULSES IN AMPUTATED PATIENTS								
AMPUTATION	POSTERIOR TIBIAL*				DORSALIS PEDIS*			
	Present	%	Absent	%	Present	%	Absent	%
MAJOR (n=12)	7	58.3	5	41.7	4	33.3	8	66.7
MINOR (n=41)	37	90.2	4	9.8	32	78.0	9	22.0
Total (n=53)	44	83.0	9	17	36	68.0	17	32.0

*By clinical palpation and hand Doppler.

TABLE 16: RISK FACTORS FOR LEA IN PATIENTS WITH DIABETIC FOOT ULCERS					
RISK FACTORS	AMPUTATION (n=53)		NON AMPUTATION (n=67)		P value	SIGNIFICANCE
	No. Of Patients	%	No. Of Patients	%		
SMOKING	37	69.8	26	38.8	0.0014	HIGHLY SIGNIFICANT
ALCOHOL	33	62.2	21	31.3	0.0014	HIGHLY SIGNIFICANT
NEUROPATHY	33	62.2	0	0	indeterminate	indeterminate
RETINOPATHY	33	62.2	0	0	indeterminate	indeterminate
NEPHROPATHY	26	49.0	0	0	indeterminate	indeterminate
DURATION Of DIABETES > 5 years	44	83.0	34	50.7	0.00049	HIGHLY SIGNIFICANT
OSTEOMYLELITIS	27	50.9	0	0	indeterminate	indeterminate
GENDER(MALE)	38	71.7	35	52.2	0.0301	SIGNIFICANT
PVD(ABPI<0.9)	51	96.2	46	68.7	0.00035	HIGHLY SIGNIFICANT

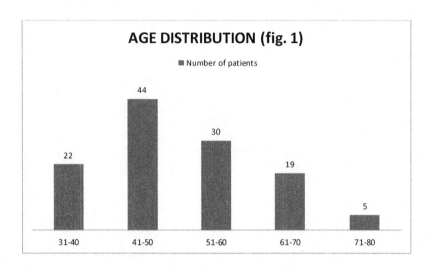

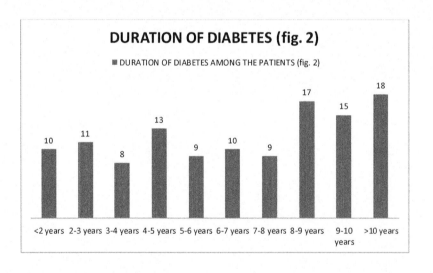

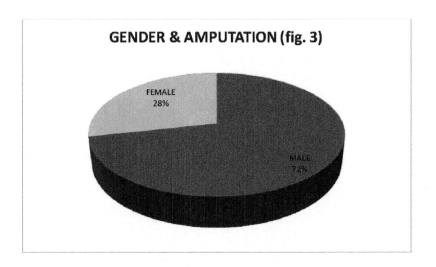

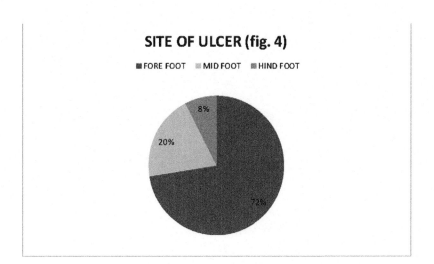

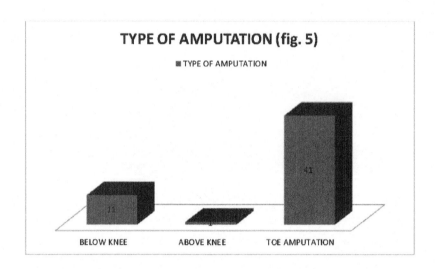

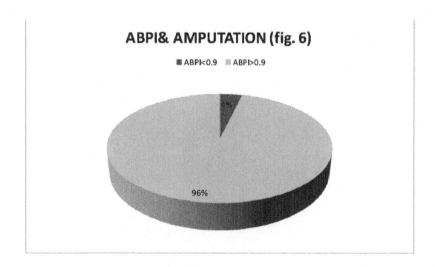

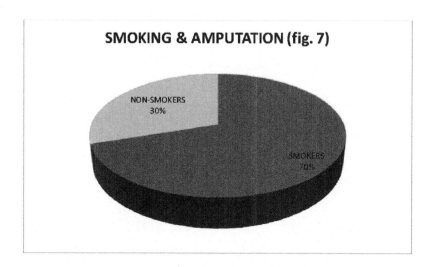

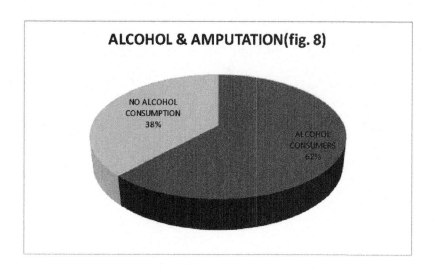

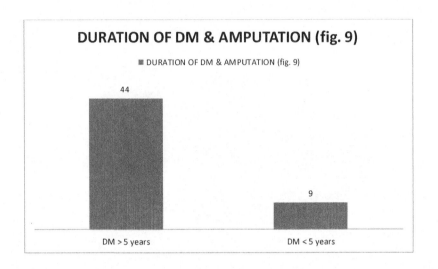

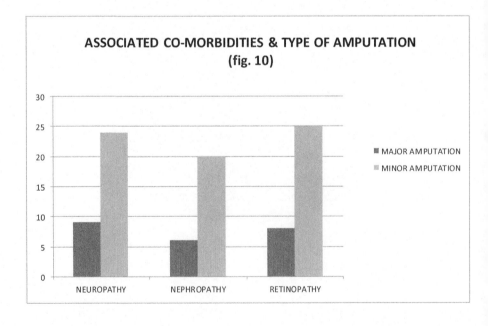

DISCUSSION

Foot infection in persons with diabetes is a common (20% of all hospital admissions of diabetic patients), complex and a costly problem [86]. In addition to causing severe morbidities, they now account for the largest number of diabetes-related hospital bed days (as long as 26 weeks for full recovery) [87] and are most common non traumatic cause for amputation (6 per 1000) [88]. Observational studies suggest that 6-43% patients of diabetes and a foot ulcer eventually progress to amputation [87, 89]. Ramsey et al. [90] reported amputation rates of 11.2% in patients with new onset foot ulcers over a 4-year period. *In our study, 53 of the 120 patients (44.17 %) studied underwent amputation and is in accordance with the reported rates in literature.*

The main underlying risk factors for foot ulcers in diabetic patients are peripheral neuropathy and ischemia. The primary goal in the treatment of diabetic foot ulcer is to treat the ulcer and save the limb from amputation. The single most important factor in preventing amputation is detailed and repeated education of the patient in foot care.

The incidence of diabetic foot increases with increase age group [48, 49, 57, 65, 72, 76]. Many studies revealed that the mean age group was in the 6th and 7th decade.

Al-Maskari et al studied the prevalence of risk factors for diabetic foot complications. Out of 513 diabetic patients (mean age of 53 years) 39% had peripheral neuropathy and 12% had peripheral vascular disease. Significant risk factors were male gender, poor level of education, increased duration of diabetes and presence of hypertension [49].

Al-Tawfiq from Saudi Arabia evaluated the presentation and outcome of diabetic foot ulcers in Saudi Arabian patients. Out of 62 patients (mean age 64.8 years) all patients with diabetic foot ulcers of Wagner grade 4 or 5, hypertension, peripheral vascular disease, absence of pedal pulses and ischemic heart disease underwent amputation [57].

Mehamud et al.[48] of Pakistan in his paper, 'clinical profile, management and outcome of diabetic foot ulcers in tertiary care hospital', determined that out of 120 patients, majority of patients who underwent amputation had type 2 diabetes (95.7%), males (66%), with duration of diabetes more than 10 years (p<0.05). The mean age was 54.29 +/- 7.71 years. Male gender is a significant risk factor for amputation [48, 49, 57]. In our study we found that the highest incidence was in the 5th decade (36.7%) and 60.8% were males. Male gender was at significantly higher risk for lower extremity amputation (P: 0.0301).

The duration of diabetes also plays a role in the formation of ulcer and the incidence of lower extremity amputation was more in patients who have diabetes for more than 5 years [19, 50, 51,58,65,68].

Krittiyawong et al. studied the prevalence and the risk factors associated with lower extremity amputation in Thai diabetics. This cross sectional study revealed that the mean duration of diabetes was 10 years, of the 556 patients, 370 who had peripheral vascular disease (PVD) (64.1%) underwent toe amputations. Multiple logistic regression analysis of the risk factors revealed a high risk of lower extremity amputation in peripheral vascular disease, diabetic retinopathy and in patients with diabetes for longer than 10 years[50].

Leelawattana et al. in her project of prevalence of vascular complication in long standing type 2 diabetes described that the complications were amputation (5.5%), stroke (9.4%), and foot ulcer (13.4%). The project involved 9284 patient of which 2244 were of long standing type 2 diabetics-mean duration 7.0+/-3.9 years [51].

Similarly in our study, out of 120 patients 78 patients had diabetes for more than 5 years. 44 patients underwent amputation. This was statistically significant risk factor for lower extremity amputation (P value: 0.00049)

Male gender is at increased risk factor amputation ([48, 49,61,69,71, 81]).

A case control study of the risk factors for toe amputation in a diabetic population by Carlson et al showed that the obvious risk factors for toe amputation were male sex, osteomyelitis digital deformity, diabetic nephropathy, neuropathy, and ischemia[61].

Risk factors associated with adverse outcomes in a population based prospective cohort study of people with their first diabetic foot ulcer by Winkley et al of UK explained the variables were age, male gender, smoking, ulcer site, size, severity of neuropathy, ischemia, HbAlc levels, presence of vascular complications. In a group of 253 patients 36 patients had amputations (15.5%). Microvascular complications were the only explanation for recurrent ulceration[81]. Out of 120 patients in our study 73 were males and 38 patients had amputation. Male gender was at significantly higher risk for lower extremity amputation (P: 0.0301).

Amputation rate is higher in type 2 diabetics.

Alwakeel et al. studied concomitant macro and microvascular complications in diabetic nephropathy. Out of 1952 type 2 diabetic patients the mean age was 66.9+/-11.4 years, mean duration of diabetes was 15.4+/-7.5 years, the mean age of onset of nephropathy was 61.5+/-12.4 years and the mean duration of nephropathy was 3.9+/-3.8 years. The complications were limb amputation (3.7%), retinopathy (11.7%), peripheral neuropathy (24.9%), myocardial infarction (24.1%), and acute coronary syndrome (36.1%). The relative risk of developing these complications was significant after the onset of nephropathy[65].

A fourfold increase in foot ulcers in type2 diabetic subjects without an increase in major amputation by a multidisciplinary setting was a review from Denmark by Hedetoft et al. The end result was neuropathy and ischemia were important risk factors for amputation (p<0.05)[66].

Other studies by Mehmood et al, and Leelawattana et al proved that type 2 Diabetic patients were at increased risk for amputation. All of our patients were type 2 diabetics[48, 51].

The associated risk factor included smoking and consumption of alcohol. Hypertension and hyperlipidemia were the comorbidities which favored amputation. Many studies have indicated these factors as risk factors for amputation ([56, 68, 75, 81, 85]). Hypertension and hyperlipidemia was present in 86 and 98 patients respectively and were both significant risk factors for development of foot ulcers in diabetics. However, they were not statistically significant for amputation.

Chaturvedi et al. in his article of risk of diabetes – related amputation in south Asians vs. Europeans in the UK, observed a decrease by quarter in the risk of amputation in south Asians as compared with Europeans. This was explained by low rates of PVD, neuropathy, alcohol consumption and smoking in south Asians as compared with the Europeans [85].

A study of 217 patients from university of Malaya Medical Centre to evaluate the prevalence and risk factors for diabetic retinopathy by Tajunisah et al were, duration of diabetes, hypertension, presence of systemic complications (diabetic foot ulcer , lower limb amputation, nephropathy and peripheral neuropathy). The association of lower limb amputation and diabetic retinopathy was stressed in this study [68].

Our study had 63 smokers, 54 patients consuming alcohol. 69.8% and 62.2% of patients who underwent amputation were smokers and consumed alcohol respectively. They were found to be significant risk factors for amputation (P: 0.0014 for both).

Peripheral pulses monitored in our study were posterior tibial and dorsalis pedis which was present in 99 and 82 patients respectively. The absence peripheral pulses and presence of peripheral vascular disease as indicated by a low Ankle Brachial pressure index of less than 0.9, favors the formation of diabetic foot ulcer and increase the incidence of amputation. In our study, of the 53 patients who underwent amputation only 2 had ABPI>0.9 and of the 120 patients studied, only 23 had ABPI>0.9.

Dalla et al. proved that peripheral vascular disease is the only main risk factor leading to amputation. Peripheral vascular disease not only involves the distal pulses but also involves the femoral and popliteal pulses[73].

ABPI of less than 0.9 which is an outcome of peripheral vascular disease proceeds to amputation has been mentioned by Davis et al and Nather et al. In our study 51 out of 53 patients has abnormal ABPI of less than 0.9[74,75]

Several other studies also have stressed upon the relation of peripheral vascular disease and amputation.

Diabetic heel ulcers: Major risk factors for lower extremity amputation (LEA) by Younes et al. describes out of all foot ulcers seen in diabetic patients heel ulcers are the most serious and often lead to LEA. The most common risk factors for ulceration in the heel are immobility of the lower limbs, retinopathy, PVD, structural deformity, and poor foot hygiene[83].

Frykberg et al in his study of diabetic foot ulcers: pathogenesis and management in 2002 proved the most frequent etiologies are neuropathy, trauma, deformity, PVD and high plantar pressures. A multidisciplinary management is needed that focuses on prevention, patient education , regular foot examination, optimal use of therapeutic foot wear has reduced the incidence of LEA[84].

Krittyawong, Leelawattana, Miyajima and Peters et al. have also stressed on the importance of peripheral vascular disease in amputation [50, 51, 52, 53]

Neuropathy is considered if three of the following four sensations were absent, light touch, pain, vibration and tendon reflexes. The risk for amputation is higher with PVD than that for neuropathy [91]. Distinction between neuropathic and vascular ulcers is not a clear one, because neuropathy may contribute to foot ulceration via effects on the microcirculation. Lavery et al. claimed that neuropathy, but not vasculopathy, in the patients with diabetes was a risk factor for ulcers [80]. It is plausible that neuropathy may precipitate an ulcer and vasculopathy may prevent its healing. In our study 51 out of 53 patients who underwent amputation had PVD (ABPI less than 0.9). We found that ABPI<0.9 (PVD) was a statistically significant risk factor for amputation (0.00035). This finding emphasizes the importance of PVD and its significance to LEA.

The most frequently cultured microorganism in our study was Proteus species (26.7%), followed by E.coli (20.8%). Polymicrobial infection was present in 19.2 % of patients. But polymicrobial infection is associated with diabetic foot ulcers, as reported in literature [77, 78]. This change could be attributed to local flora of the place.

Risk assessment of the diabetic foot and wound by Wu et al in 2005 stated the key factors associated with the non-healing of diabetic foot wound and therefore amputation include wound depth, presence of polymicrobial infection and presence of ischemia[82].

Of all the complications peripheral Neuropathy is the most important factor in the formation of ulcers and leading to amputation. Al-Maskari et al proved (39%) of his patients had neuropathy[49].

Elliot et al analyzed that large fibre dysfunction in diabetic peripheral neuropathy is predicted by cardiovascular risk factors. Large fibre dysfunction as measured by vibration perception threshold predicts foot ulceration, amputation and mortality. Vibration perception threshold (VPT) was measured by biothesiometry on 1407 patients with mean duration diabetes 14.7+/-9.3 years mean age of 32.7+/-10.2 years. The result was abnormal VPT had increased the incidence of amputation. VPT was influenced by duration of diabetes, high HbAlc, male sex (p=0.0004), hypertension (p<0.0001), smoking (p<0.0001), total cholesterol (p=0.01), and diabetic retinopathy nephropathy (p=0.001)[58].

Casellini et al also proved that involvement of small nerve fibres causes neuropathy and that large fibres cause ataxia, incoordination and falls[59]. Peters and Alder et al. also reported neuropathy to be a major cause for amputation[53, 55].

Vishwanathan et al. elaborated that 15% of his amputated patients had neuropathy. Hennis, Tajunisah, Bartus, Lavery and Frykberg et al have emphasized on the presence of neuropathy as an associated risk for lower extremity amputation [60, 63, 68, 70, 80, 84].

Retinopathy and nephropathy also indicate that the duration of diabetes has been long enough to cause significant damage to the end organs. It also proves that there is poor glycemic control in these patients.

Margolis et al. compared the association between renal failure and foot ulcer or lower extremity amputation in patients with diabetes. The study proved that there is a strong association between chronic kidney disease and diabetic foot ulcer irrespective of the presence or absence of peripheral disease. Patients even with moderate chronic kidney disease (<60ml/min per 1.73 m2) had an increased risk of diabetic foot ulcer or lower extremity amputation[54].

Retinopathy is a risk factor which favors amputation[56, 68]. The Wisconsin epidemiologic study of diabetic retinopathy of 14 year incidence of lower extremity amputation is diabetic patients concluded high blood pressure, history of ulcers, more severe retinopathy high glycosylated hemoglobin were significant risk factors for lower extremity amputation[56].

Neuropathy, retinopathy and nephropathy if present in a patient most often proceed towards amputation. In our study, 33 out of 53 amputations had neuropathy and retinopathy. Nephropathy was present in 26 patients out of 53 patients. These numbers show that they were closely related to amputation. However, the P value could not be determined as none of the patients in the non-amputation group had these complications. The same was found with osteomyelitis. 50.9% patients who underwent amputation had associated osteomyelitis, but the P value could not be determined for the same reason stated above.

Revascularization helps in salvaging the limb amputation.

Faglia et al in his prospective study of peripheral angioplasty (PTA) as the first choice revascularization procedure in diabetic patients with critical limb ischemia evaluated 993 patients who underwent peripheral angioplasty. The 5 year primary patency was 88%. He proved that PTA as the first choice revascularization procedure was feasible, safe and effective for limb salvage in a high percentage of diabetic patients. Clinical re – stenosis was an infrequent event and PTA could successfully be repeated in most cases[77].

Wijeyaratnae et al. in his publication in 2003 of revascularization in diabetic small vessel disease of lower limbs: Is it worthwhile? Used saphenous vein to bypass occluded infra popliteal arteries in diabetics with critical leg ischaemia over a 5 year period on 23 patients. He noted patency in 65% of patients at a mean follow up of 30 months. He concluded that Bypass of diabetic small vessel disease of the lower limbs is feasible and effective in preventing major amputation and maintaining independent mobility [78].

In 1996 De Campo et al. from Canada in his case report on Microvascular free myocutaneous flap for treatment of non-healing ischemic ulcers of the lower extremity discovered that arterial reconstruction alone failed to stimulate healing of lesions with exposed bone and tendons in weight-bearing areas. But with a combination of percutaneous transluminal angioplasty and a microvascular free myocutaneous flap, complete healing of the ulcer was noted and flap was viable for 35 months[79].

CONCLUSION

The incidence of diabetic foot ulcers is higher in males and in the 5th decade of life. Associated Hypertension and Hyperlipidemia are statistically significant risk factors leading to foot ulcers in diabetics. Males are more prone for amputation. Smoking and Alcohol consumption and PVD (ABPI<0.9) and duration of diabetes more than 5 years are statistically significant risk factors for LEA. Statistical significance of associated complications such as neuropathy, nephropathy, retinopathy and osteomyelitis could not be determined.

This study provides information for primary care and specialist practitioners to identify diabetic patients at high risk for lower extremity amputation. Of the significant risk factors for LEA mentioned in our study, smoking, alcohol intake and PVD are preventable risk factors. It underlines the importance of health education and health promotion among the public. Diabetics have to be urged to quit smoking and alcohol consumption at the time of diagnosis of diabetes. The value of early diagnosis and management of diabetes cannot to be overemphasized as it may significantly reduce or delay the incidence of PVD.

BIBLIOGRAPHY

1)   Pryce TD: A case of perforating ulcer of both feet associated with diabetes and ataxic symptoms, Lancet, 1887; 11:11-2.

2)   Palumbo P.J., Melton III, L.J. Chapter XV, Peripheral Vascular disease and diabetes. In Diabetes in America: Diabetes data compiled in 1984, Washington, D.C., U.S. Govt. Printing Office (NIH publ. No.85-1468), 1985.

3)   Block P. The diabetic foot ulcer: a complex problem with a simple treatment approach. Mil Med. 1981; 146:644-6

4)   Smith DM, Weinberger M, Katz BP. A controlled trial to increase office visit and reduce hospitalizations of diabetic patients. J. Gen. Intern Med. 1987;232-8.

5)   Sathe SR; Managing the diabetic foot in developing countries. IDF Bulletin. 1993;38: 16-8

6)   Waugh NR: Amputation in diabetic patients: A review of rates, relative risks, and resource use, Comm. Med. 1988; 10 ; 279-88.

7)   Adler AI, Boyko EJ, Ahroni JH, Stensel V, Forsberg RC, Smith DG. Risk factor for diabetic peripheral sensory neuropathy, Diabetes Care 1997; 20: 1162-7.

8)   Harris M, Eastman R, Cowie C. Symptoms of sensory neuropathy in adults with NIDDM in the U.S. population. Diabetes Care 1993;16: 1446-52.

9)   Grunfed C. Diabetic foot ulcers; etiology, treatment and prevention. Adv. Intern. Med. 1991;37:103-32.

10)   Dyck PJ, Davies JL, Wilson DM, Service FJ, Melton LJ III, O' Brien PC. Risk factor for severity of diabetic polyneuropathy. Diabetes Care 1999;22:1479-86.

11)   Young D.S, Rosoklija G, Hays AP. Diabetic peripheral neuropathy. Semin Neurol. 1998; 18 (1): 95-104.

12)   Cameron NE, Cotter MA. Metabolic and vascular factors in the pathogenesis of diabetic neuropathy. Diabetes 1997;4 (2):S31-7.

13)   Borssen B, Bergenheim T, Lithner F. The epidemiology of foot lesions in diabetic patients aged 15-50 years. Diabet. Med 1990;7;438-44.

14)   Mayfield JA, Reiber GE, Sanders LJ. Janisse D, Pogach LM. Preventive foot care in people with diabetes. Diabetes care 1998;21:2161-77.

15)   LoGerfo FW, Coffman JD. Vascular and microvascular disease of the foot in diabetics; implications for foot care N. Engl. J. Med. 1984;311:1615-8.

16)   Rayman G, Hassan A, Tooke JE. Blood flow in the skin of the foot related to posture in diabetes mellitus. BMJ (Chin. Res. Ed) 1986;292 (6513):87-90

17)   McMillan DE Blood flow and the localization of atherosclerotic plaque. Stroke 1985 ; 16: 582-7.

18)   Apelqvist J, Agardh CD. The association between clinical risk factors and outcome of diabetic foot ulcers. Diabetes Res. Clin, Pract 1992; 18 (1):43-53.

19)   Mantey, I, Foster AV, Spencer S, Edmonds ME. Why do foot ulcers recur in diabetic patients? Diabet. Med. 1999; 16: 245-9.

20)   Krupski WC. The peripheral vascular consequences of smoking. Ann. Vasc. Surg 1991; 5(3):291-304.

21)   Muhlhauser . Cigarette smoking and diabetes: an update, Diabet, Med. 1994; 11: 336-43.

22)   Levin ME. An overview of the diabetic foot: Pathogenesis, management and prevention of lesions, Int. J. Diab. Dev. Countries 1994; 14: 39-47

23)   Sanders LJ, Frykberg RG: Charcot foot in Levin MEm O' Neal LW; Bowker JH (eds) The Diabetic foot 5th ed. 1993, CV Mosby Co., St. Louis Mo, 149-80

24) Oyibo SO, Jude EB, Tarawnch I, The effects of ulcer size and site, patient's age, sex and type of diabetes on the outcome of diabetic foot Ulcers, Diabet. Med.2001;18;133-138.

25) Levin ME, O' Neal LW; Bowker JH.(eds). Pathogenesis and management of diabetic foot lesions. The Diabetic Foot, 5th ed. 1993, St Louis, CV Mosby, 17-60.

26) Taylor Jr. LM, Porter JM. The clinical course of diabetics who require emergent foot surgery because of infection or ischaemia. J. Vasc. Surg. 1987; 6: 454.

27) Lichter SB, Allweiss P, Harley J, Clay J, et al. Clinical characteristics of diabetic patients with serious pedal infection, Metab. 1988; 37: 22-24

28) Newman LG, Waller J, Palestro CJ, et al. Unsuspected osteomyelitis in diabetic foot ulcer. JAMA. 1991; 266:1246-51.

29) Littenberg B, Mushlin Al. The diagnostic technology assessment consortium. Technetium bone scanning in the diagnosis of osteomylitis: a meta-analysis of test performance. J Gen Intern Med. 1992; 7:158-63.

30) Newman LG, Waller J, Palestro CJ, et al. Leukocyte scanning with I I IN is superior to magnetic resonance imaging in diagnosis of clinically unsuspected osteomyelitis in diabetic foot ulcers. Diabetes Care. 1992; 15;1527-30.

31) Bamberger DM, Daus GP, Gerding DN: Osteomylitis in the feet of diabetic patients: long-term results, prognostic factors, and the role of antimicrobial and surgical therapy. AM.J. Med. 1987; 833:653-60.

32) Lipsky BA, Pecoraro RE, Wheat LJ. The diabetic foot: soft tissue and bone infection. 1990; 4:409-32.

33) Liven MEm Spratt IL. "To soak or not to soak." ClinDiabetes. 1986; 4: 44-5.

34) Pecoraro RE, Ahroni JH, Boyko EJ, Stensel VL. Chronology and determinants of tissue repair in diabetic lower extremity ulcers. Diabetes, 1991; 40:1305-13.

35)   Sinacore DR, Muller MJ. Total-contact casting in the treatment of neuropathic ulcers. In Levin ME, O'Neal LW Bowker JH, eds. The Diabetic Foot 5th ed. St. Louis: St. Louis: Mosby-year Book. 1993; 259-81.

36)   Mills JL, Beckett WC, Taylor Sm. The diabetic foot: consequences of delayed treatment and referral. South MedJ. 1991; 84:970-4.

37)   LoGerfo FW; Gibbons GW, Pomposelli FB Jr. et al. Trends in the care of the diabetic foot: expanded role of arterial reconstruction. Arch , Surg. 1992;127: 617-21.

38)   Cianci P. Hunt TK. Adjunctive hyperbaric oxygen therapy in treatment of diabetic foot wounds. In Levin ME, O' Neal LW, Bowker JH, eds. The Diabetic foot. 5th ed. St. Louis: Mosby-Year Book. 1993; 305-19.

39)   Zhao L, Davidson JD, Wee SC, Roth SI and Mustoe TA. Effect of hyperbaric oxygen and growth factors in rabbit ear ischaemic ulcers. Arch. Of Surg. 1994; 129(10): 1043-9.

40)   Alvarez OM, Gilson G, Auletta MJ. Local aspects of diabetic foot ulcer care: assessment, dressings, and topical agents. In Levin ME, O' Neal LW, Bowker JH, eds. The Diabetic Foot, 5th ed, St. Louis: Mosby-Year Book, 1993; 259-81.

41)   Knighton Dr, Fiegel VD. Growth factors and repair of diabetic wounds. In Levin ME, O' Neal LW, Bowker JH, eds, The diabetic Foot, 5th ed. St. Louis; Mosby-Year Book. 1993; 247-57.

42)   Steed DL, Goslen JB, Holloway GA, Malone JM, Blunt TJ, Webster MW, Randomized prospective double-blind trial in healing chronic diabetic foot ulcers: CT-102 activated platelet supernatant, topical versus placebo. Diabetes Care. 1992; 15: 1598-604.

43)   Bentkover JD, Champion AH, Economic evaluation of alternative methods of treatment for diabetic foot ulcer patients; Cost effectiveness of platelet releasate and wound care cl8inics. Wounds, 1993; 5:207-15.

44)   Skerrett PJ, "Matrix algebra" heals life's wounds. Science, 1991; 252; 1064-6.

45)   Edmonds ME, Blundell MP, Morris ME, Cotton LT, Watkins PJ. Improved survival of the diabetic foot: The role of a specialized foot clinic, Q J Med. 1986; 60: 763-71.

46)   Malone JM, Synder M, Anderson G, Bernhard VM, Holloway GA Jr. Blunt TJ. Prevention of amputation by diabetic education. Am J.Surg. 1989; 158: 520-4.

47)   Litzelman DK, Slemenda CW, Langefeld CD, Hays LM, Welch MA, Bild DE, Ford ES, Vinicor F. Reduction oflower extremity clinical abnormalities in patients with non-insulin-dependent diabetes mellitus, Ann. Intern. Med, 1993; 119: 36-41.

48)   Mehmood K, Akhtar St, Talib A, Talib A, Abbasi B, Siraj-ul-Salekeen, Naqvi IH Clinical profile and management outcome of diabetic foot ulcers in a tertiary care hospital. J. Coll. Physicians Surg. Pak. 2008; Jul: 18(7): 408-12.

49)   Al-Maskari F, El-Sadig M. Prevalence of risk factors for diabetic foot complications. BMC. Fam. Pract.2007; 8:59.

50)   Krittiyawong S, ANagarmukos c, Benjasuratwong Y, Rawdarce P, Leelawatana R, Kosachunhanun N, Plengvidhya N, Deerochanawong C, Suwanwalaikorn S, Pratipanawatr T, Chetthakul T, Mongkolsomlit S, Bunnag P. Thailand diabetes registry project : prevalence and risk factors associated with lower extremity amputation in Thai diabe5tics. Med. Assoc. Thai. 2006; 89(1): 43 – 48.

51)   Leelawattana R, Pratipanawatr T, Bunnag P, Kosachunhanum N, Suwanwalaikorn S, Krittiyawong S, Cheetthakul T, Plengidhya N, Benjasuratwong Y, Deerochanawong C, Mongkolsomilt S, Nga mukos C, Rawdarce P. Thailland diabetes registry project: prevalence of vascular complications in long – standing type 2 diabetes. Journal of Med. Assoc. Thai. 2006; 89(1): 54-59.

52)   Miyajima S. Shiraj A. Yamamoto S, Okada N, Matushita T. Risk factors for maker limb amputation in diabetic foot gangrene patients. Diabetes Res. Clin. Pract. 2006; (3): 272-79.

53)   Peter EJ, Lavery LA, Armstrong DG. Diabetic lower extremity infection: influence of physical, psychological, and social factors. Journal of Diabetes Complications 2005; 19(2): 107-112.

54)   Margolis DJ, Hofstad O, Feldman H. Association Between Renal Failure and Foot Ulcer or Lower- Extremity Amputation in Patients with Diabetes. Diabetes care 2008; 31(7): 1331-36.

55)   Alder AI, Boyko EJ, Ahroni JH, Smith D.G. Lower – extremity amputation in diabetes. The independent effects of peripheral vascular disease, sensory neuropathy, and foot ulcers. Diabetes Care 1999; 22(7); 1029-1035.

56)   Moss SE, Klein R, Klein B.E. The 14 yr incidence of lower – extremity amputations in a diabetic population. The Wisconsin Epidemiologic study of Diabetic Retinopathy, Diabetes Care 2000; 23(3): 432 – 433.

57)   Al-Tawfiq JA , Johndrow JA, Presentation and outcome of diabetic foot ulcers in Saudi Arabian patients. Adv. Skin Wound Care 2009; 22(3):199-121.

58)   Elliott J. Tesfave S, Chaturvedi N. Gandhi RA, Stevents LK, Emery C, Fuller JH. Large fibre dysfunction in diabetic peripheral neuropathy is predicted by cardiovascular risk factors. Diabetes Care 2009; July 8.

59)   Casellini CM, Vinik AI, Clinical manifestations and current treatment options for diabetic neuropathies. Endocr. Pract ,2007; 13(5); 550-566.

60)   Viswanathan V, Thomas N, Tandon N, Asirvatham A. Rajasekar S, Ramachandran A, Senthilvasan K, Murugan VS, Muthulakshmi. Profile of diabetic foot complications and its associated complications- a multicentric study from India. Journal of Assoc. Physicians India 2005; Nov53: 933-36

61)   Carlson T, Reed JF, A case-control study of the risk factors for the amputation in a diabetic population. Int. Journal of Low. Extrem. Wounds 2003; 2(1):19-21.

62)   Van Damme H, Limet R. Amputation in diabetic patients. Clin Podiatr Med Surg 2007; 24(3): 569-582.

63)   Hennis AJ, Fraser Hs, Jonnalagadda R, Fuller J, Chaturvedi N. Explanations for the high risk factors of diabetes-related amputation in a Caribbean population of black African descent and potential for prevention. Diabetes Care 2004; 27(11):2636-41.

64)   Moss SE, Klein R, Klein BE, Wong TY, Retinal vascular changes and 20 years incidence of lower extremity amputations in a cohort with diabetes . Arch. Intern. Med. 2003; 163(20):2505-10.

65)   Alwakeel JS, Al-Suwaida A, Isnani AC, Al-Harbi A, Alam A. Concomitant macro and microvascular complications in diabetic nephropathy. Saudi Journal of Kidney Dis. Transpl. 2009; 20(3): 402-09.

66)   Hedetoft C, Rasmussen A, Fabrin J, Kolendorf K. Four-fold increase in foot ulcers in type 2 diabetic subjects without an increase in major amputations by a multidisciplinary setting. Diabetes Res. Clin. Pract 2009; 83(3):353-357..

67)   Senneville E, Infection and diabetic foot Rev. Med. Interne. 2008; 29(2):243-248

68)   Tajunisah I, Nabilah H, Reddy SC, Prevalence and risk factors for diabetic-retinopathy – a study of 217 patients from university of Malaya medical centre. Med. Journal of Malaysia 2006; 61(4):451-456.

69)   Markowitz JS, Gutterman EM, Magee G, Margolis DJ. Risk of amputation in patients with diabetic foot ulcers: a claims – based study. Wound Repair Regen, 2006; 14(1): 11-17.

70)   Bartus CL, Margolis DJ. Reducing the incidence of foot ulceration and amputation in diabetes. Curr. Diab. Rep.2004; 4(6); 413-418.

71)   Dos Santos VP, da Silverira DR, Caffaro RA. Risk factors for primary major amputation in diabetic patients. Sao Paulo Med. Journal 2006; 124(2) ; 66-70.

72)   Imran S, Ali R, Mahboob G, Frequency of lower extremity amputation in diabetics with refrence to glycemic control and Wagner's grades. J. Coll, physicians Surg. Pak. 2006; 16(2): 124-7.

73)   Dalla Paola L, Faglin E. Treatment of diabetic foot ulcer; an overview strategies for clinical approach. Curr. Diabetes Rev.2006; 2(4); 431-447.

74)   Davis Wa, Norman PE, Bruce DG, Davis TM, Predictors, consequences and costs of diabetics – related lower extremity amputation complicating type 2 diabetics; the Fremantle diabetes study, Diabetologia 2006; 49(11); 2634-2641.

75)   Nather A, Bee CS, Huak CY, chew JL, Lin CB, Neo S, Sim EY. Epidemiology of diabetic foot problems and predictive factors for limb loss. Journal of Diabetes Comlications 2008; 22(2): 77-82.

76)   Unnikrishnan AG. Approach to a patient with a diabetic foot.   National Medical Journal of India 2008; 21(4):201.

77)   Faglia E, Dalla Paola L, Clerici G, Clerissi J, Graziani L, Fusaro M, Gabrielli L, Loss S, Stella A, Gargiulo M, Mantero M, Caminiti M, Ninkovic S, Curci V, Morabito A. Peripheral angioplasty as the first-choice revascularization procedure in diabetic patients with critical limb ischemia: prospective study of 993 consecutive patients hospitalized and followed between 1999 and 2003. Cur. J. Vasc. Endovasc. Surg.2005; 29(6): 620-627.

78)   Wijeyaratne SM. Revascularisation in diabetic small vessel disease lower limbs; is it worthwhile? Ceylon Med. J. 2003; 48(1); 7-9.

79)   Del Campo C, Tovar E A. Microvascular free myocutaneous flap for treatment of nonhealing ischemic ulcers of the lower extremity. A case report. Tex. Heart Inst.J. 1996; 23(3): 222-225.

80)   Lavery LA, Peters EJ, Armstrong DG. What are the most effective interventions in preventing diabetic foot ulcers? International Wound journal 2008; 5(3):425-433.

81)   Winkley K, Stahl D, Chalder T, Edmonds ME, Ismail K. risk factors associated with adverse outcomes in a population –based prospective cohort study of people with their first diabetic foot ulcer. Journal of Diabetes Complications 2007; 21(6): 341-349.

82)   Wu S, Armstrong DG, Risk assessment of the diabetic foot and wound. International Wound journal 2005; 2(1):17-24.

83)   Younes NA. Albsoul AM, Awad H. Diabetic heel ulcers: a major risk factor for lower extremity amputation. Ostomy. Wound management 2004; 50 (6): 50-60.

84)   Fryberg RG. Diabetic foot ulcers; pathogenesis and management, American Fam. Physician 2003; 68(12):2327,2330.

85)   Chaturvedi N, Abbott CA, Whalley A, Widdows P, Leggtetter SV, Boulton AJ. Risk of diabetes-related amputation in South Asians Vs. Europeans in the UK. Diabetes Med.2002; 19(2): 99-104.

86)   Lipsky BA – A report from the international consensus on diagnosing and treating the infected diabetic foot. Diabetes Metab. Res. Rev. 2004; 20: 68-77.

87)   Reiber GE, The epidemiology of diabetic foot problems. Diabet. Med. 1996; 3:6-11.

88)   Reiber GE, Vileikyte L, Boyko EJ, et al – causal pathways for incident lower – extremity ulcers in patients with diabetes from two settings. Diabetes care 1999; 22: 157-62.

89)   Slovenkai MP: Foot problems in diabetes. Med. Clin. North. America 82:949-971, 1998

90)   Ramsey SD, Newton K, Blough D, McCuloch DK, Sandhu N, Reiber GE, Wagner EH : Incidence, outcomes, and cost of foot ulcers in patients with diabetes. Diabetes Care 22:382-387, 1999.

91)   *Amanda I. Adler, Jessie HA, Edward JB, Douglas GS: Lower-Extremity Amputation in Diabetes: the independent effects of peripheral vascular disease, sensory neuropathy, and foot ulcers. Diabetic Care, Volume 22, Number 7, July 1999.*

92)   *Sunil V. Kari. An economical way to offload diabetic foot ulcers [Mandakini Offloading device]. Ind. Jour. Surg. Volume 72, November 2010, 134-135.*

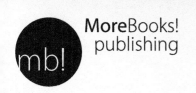
MoreBooks!
publishing

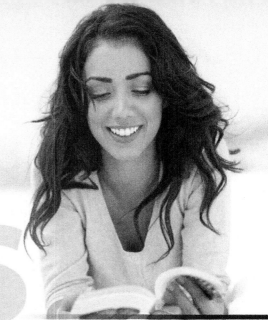

i **want** morebooks!

Buy your books fast and straightforward online - at one of world's
fastest growing online book stores! Environmentally sound due to
Print-on-Demand technologies.

Buy your books online at
www.get-morebooks.com

Kaufen Sie Ihre Bücher schnell und unkompliziert online – auf einer
der am schnellsten wachsenden Buchhandelsplattformen weltweit!
Dank Print-On-Demand umwelt- und ressourcenschonend produzi-
ert.

Bücher schneller online kaufen
www.morebooks.de

VDM Verlagsservicegesellschaft mbH
Heinrich-Böcking-Str. 6-8   Telefon: +49 681 3720 174   info@vdm-vsg.de
D - 66121 Saarbrücken   Telefax: +49 681 3720 1749   www.vdm-vsg.de

Printed in Great Britain
by Amazon

61886706R00051